THE WELLNESS

An Interactive Text

Second Edition

Thomas P. McHugh
Roscoe G. Hastings
Craig M. Rand
Monroe Community College

KE **KENDALL/HUNT PUBLISHING COMPANY**
4050 Westmark Drive   Dubuque, Iowa 52002

Copyright © 1994, 1997 by Kendall/Hunt Publishing Company

ISBN 0-7872-4182-2

Printed in the United States of America

10   9   8   7   6

CONTENTS

CHAPTER ONE
Why Physical Fitness?

Ask the next one hundred people you meet if they should be physically fit. There is almost universal agreement that everyone should be fit.

Recent studies verify that seventy percent of those surveyed said that they exercised. Of those who said they exercised only twenty percent exercised often enough, or at an intensity level that would develop or maintain an acceptable level of physical fitness.

Most people agree about the importance of physical fitness, yet the majority of Americans have inadequate levels of physical fitness. In this chapter you will learn why physical fitness is important from a physical, psychological and economic perspective.

Is Physical Fitness good for you?
__/__ Yes _____ No
Do you participate in regular exercise (Minimum of 3 times per week)?
_____ /Yes _____No

DEFINITION
There are many interpretations of what the term physical fitness means. Simply stated physical fitness is the capacity to carry out your chosen occupation successfully, enjoy your leisure time and meet an emergency if it should arise.

HISTORY
Primitive man had to be physically fit to provide food, lodging and protection for his family. The hard physical work required to provide these needs was sufficient to maintain an adequate level of physical fitness. In the last 100 years we have gone from walking for transportation to space travel. We have literally made every task that we encounter physically easier. The result is that, in most cases, an adequate level of fitness can no longer be maintained by our occupations. It is because of this, that the physical fitness level for most people has deteriorated in recent years.

List two ways that your job as a student is easier today than it was for students 100 years ago.

1. *Internet - ~~too~~ lesser need to go to library*
2. *Car - drive to school*

During this period of time, the great rise in technology has enabled us to provide vaccines that have greatly reduced the death rates from infectious diseases. Some examples of infectious diseases are measles, mumps, polio and small pox. In 1977 small pox was totally eliminated world wide. At the same time the prevalence of hypokinetic disease has risen rapidly. Hypokinetic diseases are those diseases that result from reduced physical activity. They include cardiovascular disease, hypertension, obesity, anxiety, depression and low back problems. We have become the victims of a highly technical, overindulgent, emotionally stressful and affluent society.

How many people do you know who have polio?
Zero

The physical needs of the human body are the same today as they were for primitive man. The reason is simple. The body thrives on physical activity. When exercised it becomes strong and efficient. When deprived of exercise it becomes weak and ineffective.

In today's society we have to make exercise an additional part of our daily routine. Physical fitness can no longer be achieved during our working hours. Regular exercise sessions can provide us with improved physical capacity, improved health, improved mental health and significant economic benefits.

How many people do you know who have had a heart attack or heart surgery?
too many

PHYSICAL BENEFITS

Research has shown that physical activity improves the physical functioning of the human body. Physical tasks can be performed more readily and with less fatigue. The following are specific benefits that result from adequate physical activity.

- Increased muscle tone, strength, flexibility and endurance.
- Increased ability to take in, circulate and use oxygen.
- Greater work capacity.
- Reduced muscle fatigue.
- Greater work efficiency.
- Faster recovery after vigorous exertion.
- Lower heart rate.
- Delay in the aging process.

Research also has shown that physical activity is a benefit by reducing the impact of illness and injuries. The maintenance of adequate fitness levels has demonstrated the following results:

- Decreased risk of developing or dying from chronic diseases.
- Reduced risk of Coronary Heart Disease. The least active people are twice as likely to suffer heart disease as are active people.
- Reduced risk of death. The Harvard Alumni study indicates that sedentary people who have become active have reduced their risk of death by 24 percent.
- Improved chance of surviving a heart attack.
- Decreased risk of developing infectious diseases.
- Stronger muscles reduce the risk of injuries.
- Greater flexibility reduces joint sprains.
- Reduced risk of low back injuries.
- Maintenance of body weight.
- Decreased recovery time after injuries, illness and child birth.
- Reduced impact of osteoporosis.

PSYCHOLOGICAL BENEFITS

Most people start an exercise program for health reasons. After a few months of regular exercise if you ask these people why they exercise most will tell you, "because it makes me feel good." This is one example of the psychological benefits of exercise. Activity that has the intensity to provide for the development or maintenance of fitness must be hard physical work. When one completes an easy task there is little reward, but having completed a difficult task provides for a sense of accomplishment or a "good feeling." When you motivate yourself to undertake and complete a difficult task there is a great sense of self satisfaction. Thus the performance of physical activity can improve one's self esteem. This improved vision of self worth changes one's outlook on all phases of their life.

Why do most people start an exercise program?
Health reasons

The release of catecholamines or beta-endorphins by the brain provide for what is often referred to as the runner's high. These chemicals act as pain killing drugs and can provide a euphoric state.

Stress is an internal physical reaction to our environment. Exercise can divert attention from stress producing thoughts.

The following are some psychological benefits attributed to exercise.

- Increased ability to cope with stress.
- Increased ability to resist depression.
- Improved ability to convey emotional needs to others.
- Improved physical appearance that psychologically impacts one's self esteem.
- Better relaxation and sleep patterns.
- Physical activity provides greater relief from mental stress than either valium or alcohol and without the accompanying side effects.

ECONOMIC BENEFITS

The cost of medical care in the United States rose from $97.2 billion in 1984 to $496.6 billion in 1987. Absenteeism and employee turnover are currently two of the most critical problems that U.S. industry faces. According to Johns, absenteeism costs U.S. industry $30 billion per year. Citibank put a price tag on health care of $1,936 per employee. It was projected that in 1982 the cost of each General Motors automobile included $480 for health care for their employees. The continued upward spiral of health care costs increases the price that we must pay for every product or service.

Cardiovascular disease accounts for fifty percent of all deaths in the U.S. Heart attacks cost industry 132 million workdays lost each year. This is not just a disease of the elderly. Seventy percent of servicemen, ages 22 or less, killed in Korea and Viet Nam had the beginning stages of atherosclerosis.

According to U.S. National Safety Council data, low back problems cost American industry a billion dollars in lost goods and services and 225 million dollars in workman's compensation payments.

The Rand Corporation study indicates that individuals who choose a sedentary lifestyle impose a lifetime subsidy of $1,900 on the rest of society. It should be noted that the cost would be considerably higher, were it not for the fact that sedentary individuals die earlier, and therefore receive less in pensions and social security payments.

Dr. Roy Shephard calculated that industry can save $513 per employee per year with the implementation of a fitness program. The result of improved productivity, reduced absenteeism, reduced employee turnover, fewer injuries, reduced insurance premiums is reduced prices to the consumer.

SUMMARY

Sport skills have often been mistaken for physical fitness. Physical fitness can provide the physical capacity for every person to be productive in their occupation, enjoy leisure time activities and meet emergencies that arise.

Technology developed during the past 100 years has made all occupational tasks easier. We have become a "throw away" society where products and containers are used once and discarded. The human body is not a "throw away" item. You will have to use your body for 70 or more years.

You can't throw it away and get a new one. You will benefit by keeping your body in good operating condition. It thrives on activity and atrophies with disuse. Regular exercise sessions should be scheduled to maintain your level of fitness. A good level of fitness not only will improve performance in physical tasks but also allow one to achieve their maximum potential mentally. Inactive people often lack the stamina to enjoy many of the options available to them.

Regular exercise will result in both the body and mind becoming stronger and less susceptible to illness and injury. It also provides for more rapid recovery when illness or injury do occur. In many cases it will add years to your life. More importantly it will add an improved quality to your life.

The final point is that the responsibility for your physical fitness is your's alone. If you are to develop or maintain your physical fitness, it will be because you make that decision, and you do the work necessary to accomplish success.

Name ___Ryan Eller___   Grade _____

WORKSHEET 1–A

Chapter One—Why Physical Fitness?

True/False
Put the word "true" next to the benefit if it is a proven outcome of improved physical fitness levels.
Put the word "false" if it is not.

1. Hypokinetic diseases result from inactivity.   1. T
2. Hypertension is one form of hypokinetic disease.   2. T
3. A regular exercise program results in fewer days absent from work.   3. T
4. A regular exercise program can make you live longer.   4. F
5. A regular exercise program does not improve mental health.   5. F
6. The majority of adult Americans have superior levels of fitness.   6. F
7. Primitive man needed very good fitness levels for simple survival.   7. T
8. Modern man's fitness levels have become a victim of technological advancements.   8. T
9. Increased muscle strength and endurance.   9. T
10. Greater work capacity.   10. T
11. Improve oxygen efficiency.   11. T
12. Cure for cancer.   12. F
13. Cure for the common cold.   13. F
14. Stops the aging process.   14. F
15. Reduction of fatigue.   15. T
16. Prevents heart attacks.   16. F
17. Reduces the risk of having an heart attack.   17. T
18. Improved flexibility.   18. T
19. Prevents AIDs.   19. F
20. Helps maintain body weight.   20. T
21. Helps coping with stress.   21. T
22. Eliminates stress from your life.   22. F
23. Reduces the frequency of bouts of depression.   23. T
24. Enhances self esteem.   24. T
25. Prevents suicides.   25. F
26. Enhances sleep patterns.   26. T
27. Enhances relaxation.   27. T
28. Decreased levels of fitness result in more trips to the doctor.   28. T
29. Decreased levels of fitness contribute to back problems.   29. T
30. Decreased levels of fitness contribute to cardiovascular problems.   30. T
31. Decreased risk of developing a chronic disease.   31. T
32. Improved chance of surviving of heart attack.   32. T
33. Reduces the flexibility of the joints.   33. F
34. Faster recovery time from illnesses and injuries.   34. T
35. Slows down the process of osteoporosis.   35. F
36. Reduces the use of chemical "pain killers".   36. T
37. Cardiovascular disease accounts for 25% of all U.S. fatalities.   37. T

38. Back problems account for over a billion dollars in lost productivity in U.S.   38. T
39. Results in less absenteeism from work.   39. T
40. Reduced employee turnover.   40. T
41. Reduced insurance premiums.   41. T
42. Sport skills are the same as physical fitness.   42. T
43. Senior citizens cannot improve fitness levels.   43. F
44. Women cannot improve fitness levels the same as men.   44. F
45. Children are too young to improve fitness levels.   45. F
46. One kind of fitness program is best for everybody.   46. F
47. Once gained, fitness improvements are permanent.   47. F
48. Quality of life enhancement is a major benefit of fitness.   48. T
49. Fitness will always make women's thighs thin.   49. F
50. Fitness will always flatten the stomach.   50. F

Name _____ Grade _____

WORKSHEET 1-B

Chapter One—Monroe Community College Wellness Survey

Select the word that best represents your current lifestyle in response to the statement. Write the points assigned to that word in the "Points" column. Total all of the points and refer to the chart to get an interpretation of your current lifestyle with respect to the risk of accident or illness.

Key: A—Always; RG—Regularly; S—Sometimes; RR—Rarely; N—Never.

Statement

1. I speed when I am driving.
   A—5; RG—4; S—3; RR—2; N—1
2. I wear a seat belt when in a car.
   A—1; RG—2; S—3; RR—4; N—5
3. I drive after drinking alcohol.
   A—5; RG—4; S—3; RR—2; N—1
4. I ride with drivers who have been drinking.
   A—5; RG—4; S—3; RR—2; N—1
5. I keep the doors locked when traveling in a motor vehicle.
   A—1; RG—2; S—3; RR—4; N—5
6. I smoke cigarettes.
   A—5; RG—4; S—3; RR—2; N—1
7. I use smokeless tobacco.
   A—5; RG—4; S—3; RR—2; N—1
8. My normal living environment is smokefree.
   A—1; RG—2; S—3; RR—4; N—5
9. I drink more than two alcoholic beverages daily.
   A—5; RG—4; S—3; RR—2; N—1
10. I smoke marijuana daily.
    A—5; RG—4; S—3; RR—2; N—1
11. I use cocaine products daily.
    A—5; RG—4; S—3; RR—2; N—1
12. I currently use anabolic steroids or other illegal performance enhancement supplements.
    A—5; RG—4; S—3; RR—2; N—1
13. I engage in unprotected sexual activities with multiple partners.
    A—5; RG—4; S—3; RR—2; N—1
14. I get enough sleep.
    A—1; RG—2; S—3; RR—4; N—5
15. I get enough rest and relaxation.
    A—1; RG—2; S—3; RR—4; N—5
16. I engage in social activities.
    A—1; RG—2; S—3; RR—4; N—5
17. I can play and have fun.
    A—1; RG—2; S—3; RR—4; N—5
18. I am impatient.
    A—5; RG—4; S—3; RR—2; N—1
19. I get angry easily and often.
    A—5; RG—4; S—3; RR—2; N—1

Points
1. RG 4
2. S 3
3. A 5
4. N 1
5. RG 4
6. A 1
7. N 1
8. RG 4
9. N 5
10. 4
11. 1
12. N 1
13. N 1
14. 3
15. 3
16. 2
17. 1
18. 3
19. 3

50

7

20. I treat people politely and with respect.
    A—1; RG—2; S—3; RR—4; N—5   20. ___1___

21. I blame others for my misfortunes/failures.
    A—5; RG—4; S—3; RR—2; N—1   21. ___1___

22. I accept responsibility for my behavior.
    A—1; RG—2; S—3; RR—4; N—5   22. ___1___

23. I allow other people to trigger an emotional response from me.
    A—5; RG—4; S—3; RR—2; N—1   23. ___3___

24. I eat a lot of fresh fruits and vegetables.
    A—1; RG—2; S—3; RR—4; N—5   24. ___3___

25. I eat a lot of fatty and processed foods.
    A—5; RG—4; S—3; RR—2; N—1   25. ___3___

26. I eat the correct volume of food.
    A—1; RG—2; S—3; RR—4; N—5   26. ___3___

27. I drink enough water.
    A—1; RG—2; S—3; RR—4; N—5   27. ___3___

28. My body fat percentage is acceptable.
    A—1; RG—2; S—3; RR—4; N—5   28. ___2___

29. I engage in roller coasting diets. (Continuous weight gain and loss)
    A—5; RG—4; S—3; RR—2; N—1   29. ___5___

30. I use "over the counter" diet products.
    A—5; RG—4; S—3; RR—2; N—1   30. ___1___

31. I exercise at least 3 days each week.
    A—1; RG—2; S—3; RR—4; N—5   31. ___1___

32. My blood pressure is under 120/80.
    A—1; RG—2; S—3; RR—4; N—5   32. ___1___

33. My cholesterol level is under 240.
    A—1; RG—2; S—3; RR—4; N—5   33. ___1___

34. When lifting heavy objects I use good posture, lifting with my legs.
    A—1; RG—2; S—3; RR—4; N—5   34. ___3___

35. I include cardiovascular exercise in my workouts.
    A—1; RG—2; S—3; RR—4; N—5   35. ___3___

36. I dress appropriately for the exercise that I engage in. (Weight belt, proper
    foot wear, cool clothing)   36. ___1___
    A—1; RG—2; S—3; RR—4; N—5

37. I pay attention to my body and stop exercising when I become fatigued or suffer pain. 37. ___2___
    A—1; RG—2; S—3; RR—4; N—5

38. I keep a log of my workouts.
    A—1; RG—2; S—3; RR—4; N—5   38. _____

39. I follow the "no pain, no gain" philosophy of exercise.
    A—5; RG—4; S—3; RR—2; N—1   39. ___1___

40. I warm-up and cool-down when I exercise.
    A—1; RG—2; S—3; RR—4; N—5   40. ___3___

TOTAL _____

Rating Scale

40 - 71	Low Risk
72 - 103	Below Average Risk
104 - 135	Average Risk
136 - 167	Above Average Risk
168 - 200	High Risk

Name _____ Grade _____

WORKSHEET 1C—GOALS

1. _____

2. _____

3. _____

4. _____

5. _____

CHAPTER TWO

Definition of Terms

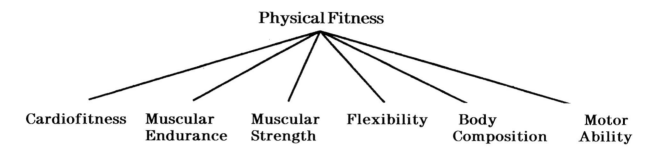

Physical Fitness

Cardiofitness · Muscular Endurance · Muscular Strength · Flexibility · Body Composition · Motor Ability

Physical Fitness is a general term used to describe the human capabilities that are physical in nature. It is defined by its components. For a person to be completely physically fit, he/she would have to address each one of the components individually.

Consequently there is no one form of training or exercise that will make a person physically fit. In order for a person to be physically fit, he/she must have a program that addresses all the components. There is no "Universal Donor" in physical fitness.

The following is a list of the components of Physical Fitness and their definitions:

Cardiofitness: The ability to take in, process, and deliver oxygen to the cells, while simultaneously eliminating waste products.
Muscular Endurance: The ability of skeletal muscle to continue to repeat an action.
Muscular Strength: The maximum amount of force or torque applied one time.
Flexibility: The ability to move a body part through a range of motion.
Body Composition: The relationship of lean, productive tissue versus fat, non-productive tissue in the body.
Motor Ability: It is a general term in itself used to describe the skill or athletic components of physical fitness.

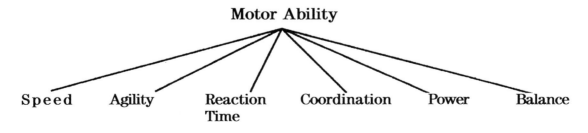

Motor Ability

Speed · Agility · Reaction Time · Coordination · Power · Balance

Motor ability refers to the skill aspect of fitness. For example, when people are watching an athlete play his or her sport, they are watching someone displaying their motor ability. Whether that athlete is physically fit is not really known at the time. The playing of the sport evaluates the athlete's skill not his/her fitness levels. Granted some sports require higher levels of fitness, but also there are some sports that require little in the nature of conditioning.

Playing sports well demonstrates superior motor ability. It doesn't demonstrate superior levels of fitness. The following is a list of components of motor ability and their definitions:

Speed: The ability to move the center of gravity of the body as fast as possible in a straight line.
(Example: Sprinter)
Agility: The ability to control the center of gravity of the body while stopping, starting and changing directions.
(Example: Running Back)
Balance: The ability to stabilize the center of gravity of the body whether moving or stationary.
(Example: Gymnast)
Reaction Time: Response time to stimulus.
(Example: Hockey Goalie)
Coordination: The integration of a number of physical skills simultaneously.
(Example: Basketball moving dribble)
Power: The ability to apply force or torque at high speeds.
(Example: Home Run Hitter)

SPECIFICITY OF TRAINING

Specificity of training simply means that there is one best way to train for each one of the components of fitness. It was previously mentioned that there is no "Universal Donor" when it comes to exercise prescriptions So the point is that one cannot achieve complete fitness by training only one way.

To achieve complete fitness, one has to train many different ways. This is the adherence to the specificity principle. For example, the runner/jogger can achieve impressive gains in cardiofitness through sound aerobic exercise prescriptions. But this aerobic exercise prescription, which was very effective for cardiofitness, contributed very little to his/her flexibility or muscular strength. Why? The answer is that the large muscle, repetitive action of aerobics is an insufficient overload to stimulate muscle strength gains. The specificity of training was not met for strength by aerobics.

Sound and effective exercise programs recognize the principle of specificity and do not allow one component to dominate the others. Inordinate emphasis on one component results in disproportionate development, which is contrary to the principles of physical fitness.

Aerobics

Aerobics simply means exercising with oxygen. It is characterized by lower intensity levels and longer durations. The aerobic exerciser will work large propulsive muscles of the body at low intensities, but for longer periods of time. Jogging, running, biking, swimming, dancing, step routines, cross country skiing, skating, and fast walking are all examples of aerobic activity. The level of intensity of work does not exceed the body's ability to deliver the oxygen. Aerobic exercise specifically improves the cardio-respiratory systems of the body.

Anaerobics

Anaerobic activity is best described as exercise bouts of high intensity but short duration. The anaerobic exerciser will work very hard for short periods of time. This type of action is most often seen in sports activities. Most sports require short bursts of highly intense action. The baseball pitching, basketball rebounding, football blocking are all examples. These short bursts are then usually followed by a drastic reduction in energy expenditure. The pitcher waiting for the signal, the foul shot in basketball, and the huddle in football often follow the intense action. Other than sports activities, some examples of this high intensity/short duration exercise would be weight lifting/power lifting and circuit training.

These exercise bouts exceed the body's ability to maintain an adequate and constant oxygen supply to the working muscles, so they are by nature time limited. The body will go into oxygen debt, and activity will soon cease. Anaerobic activity stresses the skeletal muscle system and will most likely improve its endurance and strength capabilities.

Circuit Training

Circuit training uses individual stations of resistance training equipment arranged in a circular pattern. Each piece of equipment addresses a different body part, and the user simply goes from station to station following a preset traffic pattern using slow reps of heavy resistance. The resistance equipment can be free weights, weight stack machines, pneumatic machines or hydraulic machines. Circuit training addresses the skeletal muscle system and is designed to improve the strength, endurance and flexibility of skeletal muscle.

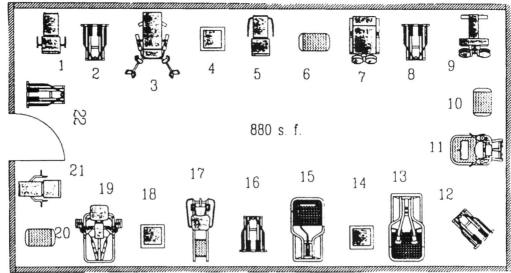

HYDRAFITNESS PACE AEROBIC CIRCUIT TRAINING

Aerobic Circuit Training

Aerobic circuit training is very similar to circuit training in that individual stations are arranged in a preset pattern. The user simply follows the traffic pattern and does a different exercise/body part at each station. The major difference between the two programs is that the latter program is timed, and the user is encouraged to exercise at a faster pace to provide a constant stress on the cardiorespiratory systems as well as the musculoskeletal system.

The exerciser will use high speed reps done with reduced resistance, while moving from station to station quickly.

Body Building

Body building is an internationally recognized form of competition that has as its primary objective the extreme development of skeletal muscle in combination with very low body fat percentages. Body building is a form of competition. It is not a form of training. Definition, symmetry, separation and vascularity are all very important objectives of the body builder. In the competition the body builder displays his/her physique development to a panel of judges who then determine who the next "Mr. America" is for example. Competitive body building requires an extreme degree of dedication. It demands daily, intense workouts of many hours each.

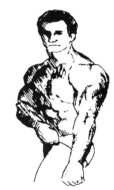

Power Lifting

Power lifting is not a form of training. It is a form of competition that has as its primary objective the lifting of the most weight possible in predetermined actions. The participants are organized into body weight classes and they compete against each other. The person who lifts the most total weight in the predetermined "lifts" is the winner. The power lifter will train with very heavy resistances and few reps. This is in contrast with the body builder who will use many sets and reps of submaximal resistance.

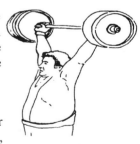

Weight Training

Weight training is a form of training and not a form of competition. The weight trainer will use some form of resistance in their exercise routine. The resistance can be free weights, or machines that have either gravity based, air, water, or hydraulic fluid resistance. Weight training programs have as their objective improvements in the strength, endurance and flexibility of skeletal muscle. There are many different exercise prescriptions for weight or resistance training, but the common denominator is that they all try to create an overload on the skeletal muscle, which serves as the stimulus for the improvement in muscle performance.

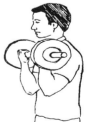

WORKSHEET 2-A

Chapter Two—Definition of Terms

Matching: Match the definition by putting the letter next to the component of fitness.

Terms/Phrases

1. Cardiofitness   1. _____
2. Muscular Endurance   2. _____
3. Muscular Strength   3. _____
4. Flexibility   4. _____
5. Body Composition   5. _____
6. Motor Ability   6. _____
7. Speed   7. _____
8. Agility   8. _____
9. Reaction Time   9. _____
10. Coordination   10. _____
11. Power   11. _____
12. Specificity of Training   12. _____
13. Balance   13. _____
14. Aerobics   14. _____
15. Anaerobics   15. _____
16. Circuit Training   16. _____
17. Aerobic Circuit Training   17. _____
18. Body Building   18. _____
19. Power Lifting   19. _____
20. Weight Training   20. _____

Definitions

A. General phrase meaning Athletic Skill.
B. Lean productive tissue related to fat non productive tissue.
C. Moving a body part through a range of motion.
D. Maximum amount of force/torque applied one time.
E. Muscle repeating action.
F. Taking in, processing and delivering O_2 while eliminating wastes.
G. Applying force/torque at high speeds.
H. Integration of a number of skills simultaneously.
I. Response time to a stimulus.
J. Stabilizing the center of gravity while moving or at rest.
K. Control center of gravity while stopping, starting or changing direction.
L. Moving center of gravity in straight line.
M. Form of training using resistance to improve strength/power.
N. Form of competition attempting to lift the most weight one time.
O. Form of competition for extreme skeletal muscle/surface anatomy development.
P. Exercising at individual stations in a preset pattern without a time limit.

Q. Exercising at individual stations in a timed and preset pattern.

R. Exercising at lower intensity for longer periods of continuous action.

S. Exercising at high intensities for short non continuous action.

T. One best way to train for each component of fitness.

CHAPTER THREE
Systems of the Body

MUSCULOSKELETAL

In order to appreciate the adaptations that occur in the human body as a result of an exercise or activity program, it is necessary to understand the involvement of the various systems of the body and their integration in that process.

SKELETAL

The skeletal system (See Fig. 3-1) is a complex system of 206 bones, each of which is best shaped to perform its primary function. Most bones are arranged in pairs on opposite sides of the body to provide skeletal symmetry. Bones are very much alive and are affected by stimuli just like any other form of living human tissue. Their performance can also be adversely affected by nutritional or boimechanical abuse.

PRIMARY SKELETAL FUNCTIONS

Levers

Long bones in the arms and legs are the levers that the human body uses to do its mechanical work. They are the mechanical tools that the muscular system uses to create human movement. Bones do not move. They are moved by the force and torque of muscle contractions.

Human Dimensions

Through heredity, the skeletal system ultimately determines the height of the person via the long bones in the legs. Also, flat bones in the shoulders and hips to a large extent determine the width of the body. Bones can also to some degree influence girth as they are the core of that particular body part. If the leg bones have a large cross sectional size, it would contribute to an overall increase in the girth of that leg.

Vital Organ Protection

Flat bones, such as the ribs or pelvis, provide protection for soft tissue vital organs via the physical block created by the hardness of the skeletal tissue. The brain and vital organs of the torso are afforded a great deal of protection from the bones surrounding them.

Joint Formation

When two or more bones come together, a joint is formed. There are over 200 joints in the body, which determine via the lever system not only the kind of movement but also the degree to which that movement occurs.

MUSCULAR SYSTEM

Muscle tissue accounts for about half of the total tissue in the body. It is the primary force for all movement of the body, whether it be the obvious action of walking or the unseen action of digestion.

There are over 600 muscles (See Figures 3-2 & 3-3), and they are divided into three different types: cardiac, smooth and skeletal. Cardiac muscle is restricted to the heart and has the single most important muscular function which is pumping blood. Smooth muscle is involuntary,which means that the person does not willfully control these actions, and is found in the vital organs.

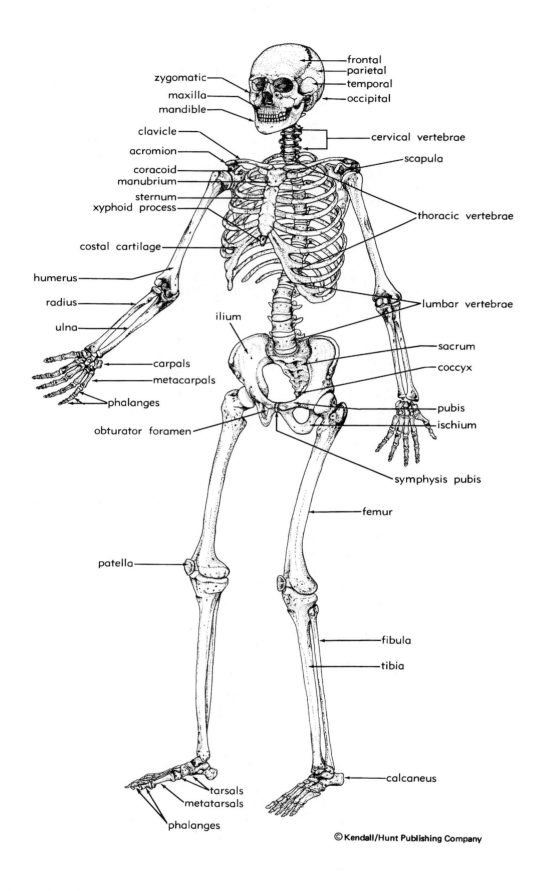

zygomatic
maxilla
mandible
frontal
parietal
temporal
occipital

clavicle
acromion
coracoid
manubrium
sternum
xyphoid process

cervical vertebrae

scapula

thoracic vertebrae

costal cartilage

humerus
radius
ulna

lumbar vertebrae

ilium

sacrum
coccyx

carpals
metacarpals
phalanges

obturator foramen

pubis
ischium

symphysis pubis

femur

patella

fibula

tibia

tarsals
metatarsals

phalanges

calcaneus

© Kendall/Hunt Publishing Company

Figure 3-1 Human Skeletal System, Ventral View (As shown)

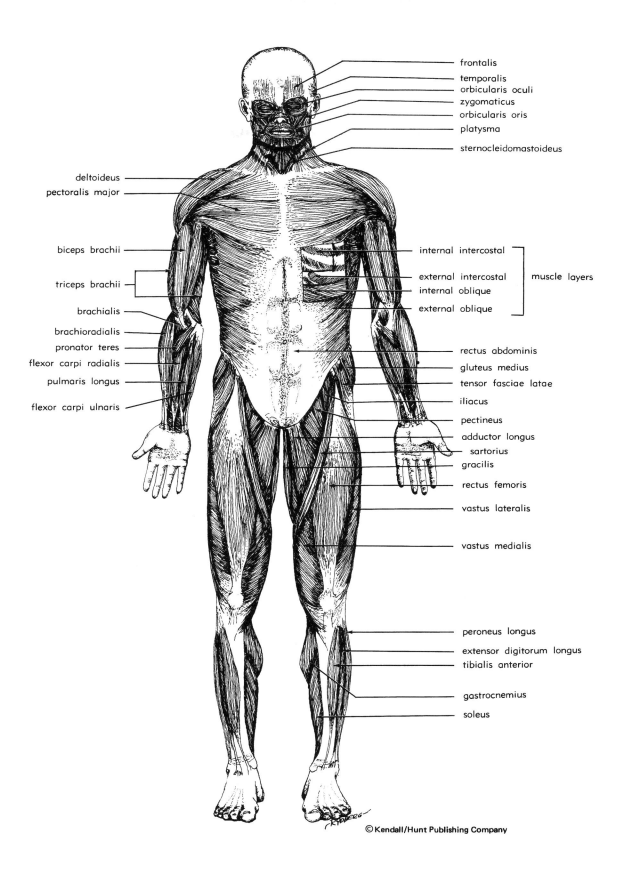

frontalis
temporalis
orbicularis oculi
zygomaticus
orbicularis oris
platysma
sternocleidomastoideus

deltoideus
pectoralis major

biceps brachii

triceps brachii

brachialis
brachioradialis
pronator teres
flexor carpi radialis
pulmaris longus

flexor carpi ulnaris

internal intercostal

external intercostal
internal oblique
external oblique

muscle layers

rectus abdominis
gluteus medius
tensor fasciae latae
iliacus
pectineus
adductor longus
sartorius
gracilis
rectus femoris
vastus lateralis

vastus medialis

peroneus longus
extensor digitorum longus
tibialis anterior

gastrocnemius

soleus

© Kendall/Hunt Publishing Company

Figure 3-2 Human Muscle System, Anterior View (As shown)

19

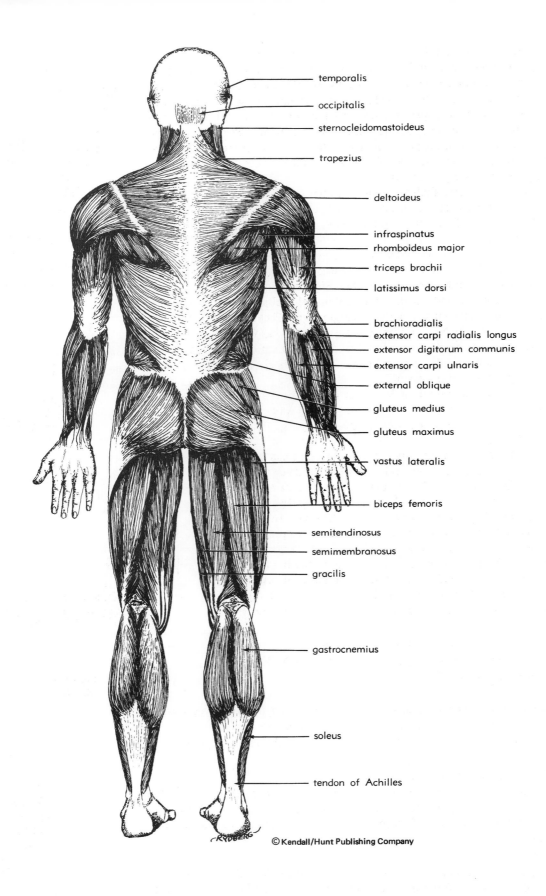

temporalis
occipitalis
sternocleidomastoideus
trapezius
deltoideus
infraspinatus
rhomboideus major
triceps brachii
latissimus dorsi
brachioradialis
extensor carpi radialis longus
extensor digitorum communis
extensor carpi ulnaris
external oblique
gluteus medius
gluteus maximus
vastus lateralis
biceps femoris
semitendinosus
semimembranosus
gracilis
gastrocnemius
soleus
tendon of Achilles

Figure 3-3 Human Muscle System, Posterior View (As shown)

The third type of muscle is skeletal, and it is responsible for all movement. It is voluntary, meaning that the individual willfully controls the action, and moves the skeleton on demand. There are over 400 skeletal muscles in the human and they range in length from inches to feet and in width from narrow strands to broad thick sheets. They are arranged in pairs on either side of the body to provide anatomical symmetry and in opposition, which means that muscles with opposite actions are located in opposite positions. This latter fact provides the balance factor for human movement. Symmetry and balance are very important considerations in all technically sound training programs.

In its simplest form, skeletal muscle is comprised of three parts: Origin Tendon, generally closest to the midline of the body; Insertion Tendon, generally farthest from the midline; and Muscle Belly, the operating structure of the muscle. (See Figure 3-4)

The tendons of the muscle attach to the bone at one end and to the muscle belly at the other. The muscle creates movement by contracting to the center, with the least stable body part moving. (See Figure 3-5)

Skeletal muscle is made up of individual muscle cells or fibers, which run longitudinally along the muscle belly (see Figure 3.6). The number of fibers per muscle is determined by the size of the muscle. The total number of muscle fibers in the body appears to be determined by heredity. The number of cells does not change as one grows and develops. The individual cells increase or decrease in size in response to the current stimuli.

Each individual cell operates independently. The more cells that are stimulated the larger the force or torque created. The entire muscle does not contract all at the same time, only the number of cells that are stimulated. This process is called recruitment. (See Figure 3-7)

Muscle fibers are broken down into two general categories, fast and slow twitch, which describes the contractile properties of these fibers. The fast twitch fibers have a high threshold for stimulation and create a large amount of force when fired. However this large force creation rapidly depletes the available energy stores creating an early onset of fatigue. The slow twitch fibers do not generate a great deal of force and are easily stimulated. This enables them to conserve energy stores and provides better endurance.

The ratio of fast to slow fibers is specific to the muscle group individually and not the body in general. Furthermore the distribution of the fibers appears to be determined by heredity and training does not appear to drastically alter their original contractile properties.

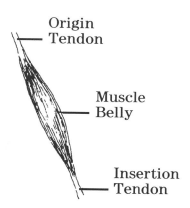

Figure 3-4 Skeletal Muscle Components

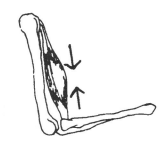

Figure 3-5 Muscle Action

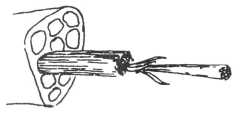

Figure 3-6 Muscle Cells

MUSCLE CONTRACTIONS

There are three types of muscle contractions: CONCENTRIC, ECCENTRIC and STATIC.

Concentric—the shortening phase of muscle contraction. It is used to overcome a resistance and occurs as the muscle fibers, which are arranged longitudinally along the muscle belly, contract and shorten. It is often called a positive contraction.

Try This Simple Demonstration

Straighten your right arm at the elbow. Place your left palm on your right bicep. Now bend your right elbow. What happened to the bicep muscle? It got shorter and thicker as the elbow became bent. This is an example of a concentric contraction.

Eccentric—the lenghtening phase of muscle contraction. It resists a force being applied to it as the fibers gradually release the concentric contraction. It is often called the negative muscle contraction.

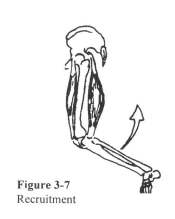

Figure 3-7 Recruitment

Try This Simple Demonstration

Retain the bent elbow position of the previous example. Put some weight in the right hand—a book, backpack handle, etc. While keeping the left hand on the right bicep, gradually lower the weight that is being held by the right hand. What happened to the right bicep? It got longer and flatter as the elbow was straightened. The concentrically contracted fibers gradually released their contraction and lengthened. This is an example of an eccentric contraction.

Static—the no movement phase of muscle contraction. It occurs when opposing pairs of muscle (Ex. Quad/Ham, Bicep/Tricep) apply equal force/torque on the lever resulting in no movement of the lever. It is the most commonly occurring contraction. It is essential in providing the support function for the skeletal system, which then allows other body parts to move.

The human body is in a continuous state of static muscle contraction unless something else assumes the support function. (Ex. Chair assumes the support function for the muscle of the legs when sitting).

NERVOUS SYSTEM

The nervous system is the ultimate determinant of skeletal muscle performance. A skeletal muscle, regardless of size or location, cannot contract to do its work unless it is stimulated by the nervous system.

The nervous system is comprised of the brain, the spinal cord and the nerve fibers that emanate from the spinal cord. There are two basic types of nerve fibers:

Sensory— which means that they pick up information and bring it back to the cord and brain.

Motor—which means that they execute the commands of the brain by stimulating the targeted muscles. This system is amazingly sensitive and complex and enables the human to have an infinite variety and degree of movement patterns.

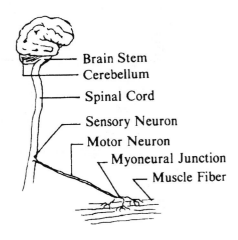

Figure 3-8 Nervous System Components

LEVER SYSTEM

The lever system is the mechanical system that the human being uses to do its work. It is comprised of three parts: the AXIS, the FORCE and the RESISTANCE.

Axis—The point around which the action occurs. The human counterpart is the joint of the body.

Force—The component that creates the work. The human counterpart is the muscle belly.

Resistance—The component that resists the work being done. The most common human counterpart is gravity.

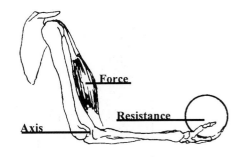

Figure 3-9 Human Lever System

WORKSHEET 3-A

Chapter Three—Label the Drawings

Muscle Components   **Nervous System**   **Lever System**

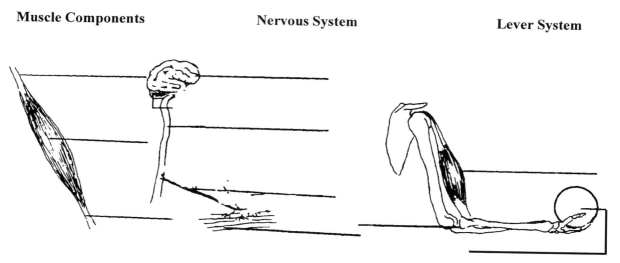

Figure 3A-1   Figure 3A-2   Figure 3A-3

Muscle Contractions—Types:

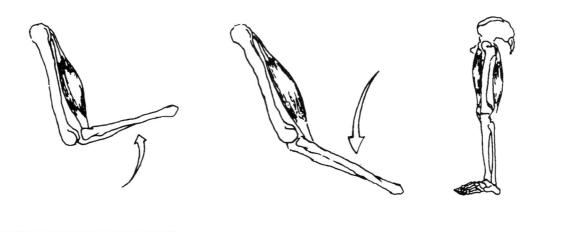

Figure 3A-4   Figure 3A-5   Figure 3A-6

CHAPTER FOUR

Systems of the Body Cardiovascular and Pulmonary

The human body is an aerobic body. The word aerobic means with air or oxygen. The human body must have a constant supply of oxygen to function. If the oxygen supply is curtailed, the cells of the body die. In this chapter you will learn about the cardiovascular system, which is a continuous circuit made up of a pump, high pressure distribution vessels, an exchange system and low pressure return vessels. You also will learn how the pulmonary system extracts oxygen from the atmosphere and makes it available to the tissues of the body for the production of energy.

> What does the word aerobic mean?
> _____

HEART

The heart is a four chamber muscular organ (See Figure 4-1) that serves as the pump providing the impetus for blood flow. The heart is about the size of your fist and weighs less than a pound. The heart, located slightly to the left of the mid-line of the body in the thoracic cavity, is composed of cardiac tissue which is similar to skeletal muscle. The difference is that cardiac muscle fibers are multinucleated, and because of their interconnecting pattern when one cell is stimulated the action potential spreads to all cells of the heart. For this reason the heart beats as a unit.

> What is the function of the human heart?
> _____

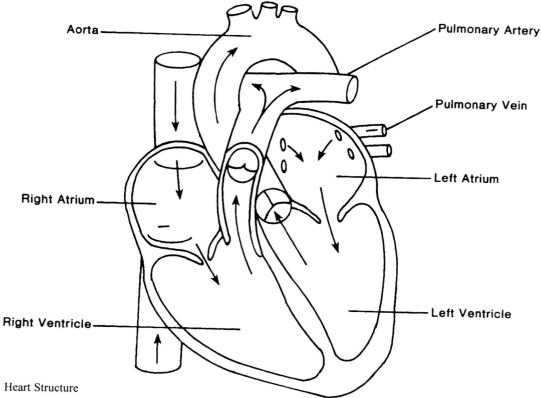

Aorta — Pulmonary Artery — Pulmonary Vein — Left Atrium — Right Atrium — Left Ventricle — Right Ventricle

Figure 4-1 Heart Structure

The four chambers fill with blood and then contract and force the blood out. The right upper chamber, right atrium, receives deoxygenated blood from the entire body. It pumps that blood to the right ventricle. The right ventricle then pumps the deoxygenated blood to the lungs via the pulmonary artery. After the exchange of gases in the lungs, the oxygen rich blood flows back to the left atrium via the pulmonary vein. The left atrium pumps the blood to the left ventricle. From the left ventricle the blood is pumped into the aorta where it is circulated to the entire body.

VASCULAR SYSTEM

The vascular system (See Figure 4-2) is the transportation network through which the blood travels throughout the body. The vessels which carry blood away from the heart are called arteries. The aorta is the large artery that carries oxygen rich blood away from the left ventricle of the heart. It branches off with arteries going to the extremities of the body. Blood traveling through the arteries has great force and travels very rapidly because of the hearts pumping force. Arteries have a pulse.

> Of what is the vascular system composed?
> _____

As the blood vessels get farther from the heart they become smaller. The smallest vessels are called capillaries. The capillaries have thin walls through which the exchange of gases occurs. Blood travels slowly through the capillaries.

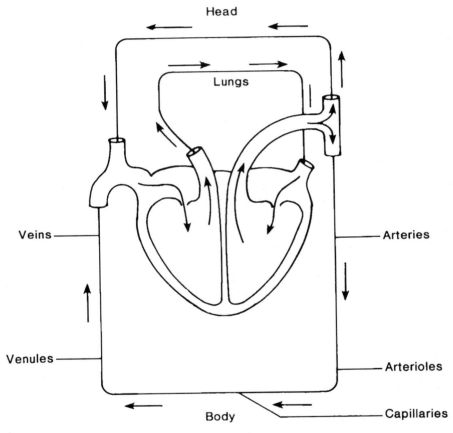

Figure 4-2 Vascular System

As the capillaries begin the return of blood to the heart they gradually become larger. They ultimately move the blood into veins. Veins are also thin walled vessels. Much of the pumping force of the heart is lost when the blood reaches the veins. The massaging action of the muscles and a system of valves helps the slow moving blood back to the right atrium of the heart. Veins carry oxygen poor blood back to the heart. The blood in the veins is a reddish brown color since it contains little oxygen. There is no pulse in the veins.

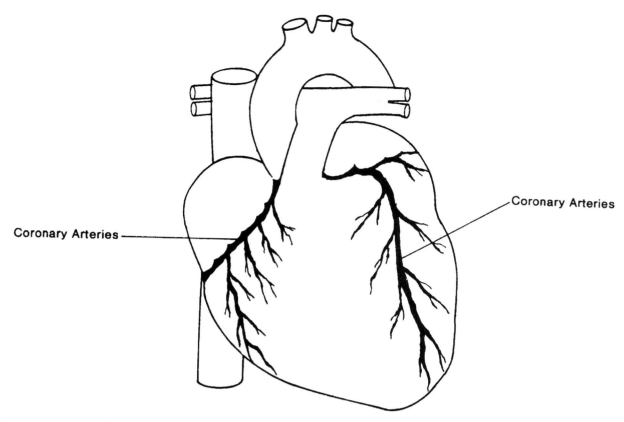

Figure 4-3 Coronary Circulation

Coronary circulation is the system of arteries, capillaries and veins that provide blood circulation to the heart muscle (See Figure 4-3) . Despite the tremendous volumes of blood flowing through the chambers of the heart, the heart muscle gets none of it's blood supply directly from the chambers. The right and left coronary arteries branch off the aorta as it leaves the heart. These arteries provide the blood supply for the heart muscle.

Blood pressure is measured in two parts. Systolic blood pressure represents the force that the left ventricle exerts in pumping the blood into the arterial system. At rest the average systolic blood pressure is 120 mm. Diastolic blood pressure provides an indication of peripheral resistance. This is an indication of the ease with which the blood flows from the arterioles to the capillaries. The average diastolic pressure is 80 mm. Blood pressure is written 120/80 with systolic on top and diastolic on the bottom.

PULMONARY SYSTEM

> What is the major organ of the pulmonary system?
> _____

The pulmonary system provides for the exchange of gases both externally and internally. The capability of this system plays a significant role in the bodies ability to function both at rest and during exercise. It is important to recognize that the system provides for the movement of gases in two directions.

The first step in pulmonary ventilation is the intake of air through the mouth and nose. In the conductive portion of the system, the air is filtered, moistened and warmed to body temperature. The air passes the trachea and moves into the two bronchi and then to the smaller bronchioles which bring it to the alveoli.

The lungs provide a surface between the blood stream and the atmospheric air. The alveoli found in the lungs are thin walled sacs. The gases, oxygen and carbon dioxide, pass through the walls of the alveoli into and out of the blood stream. This is called external respiration.

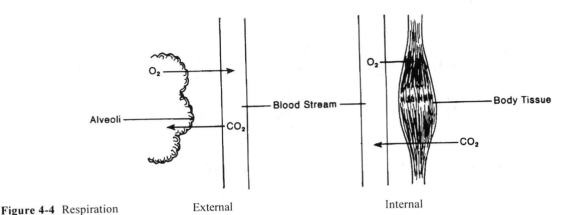

Figure 4-4 Respiration   External   Internal

Internal respiration occurs at the capillary level. Capillaries are thin walled blood vessels that allow gases to pass through to the tissues. The gases pass into and out of the tissues of the body from the capillaries.

MECHANICS OF RESPIRATION

The mechanics of breathing rely on the principles of air pressure. The principal muscle involved is the diaphragm. When it lowers, the thoracic cavity is enlarged, and air from the atmosphere rushes into the lungs until air pressure in the lungs is equal to atmospheric pressure. This is called inhalation. When the diaphragm relaxes and rises, the thoracic cavity contracts which increases the air pressure in the lungs. Air then rushes out of the lungs until atmospheric pressure equals that in the lungs. This is exhalation.

The air in the lungs contains large quantities of oxygen and small quantities of carbon dioxide. The blood in the pulmonary artery contains large quantities of carbon dioxide and small amounts of oxygen. Gases move from areas of high concentration to areas of low concentration. It is for this reason that oxygen in the lungs moves into the blood in the pulmonary artery. Carbon dioxide in the blood of the pulmonary artery moves to the lungs where it is exhaled into the atmosphere.

The blood in the capillaries contains a rich supply of oxygen. The tissues contain very little oxygen but large amounts of carbon dioxide the waste of oxidation. Again gases move from high concentrations to lower concentrations. Oxygen moves from the blood stream to the tissues where it can be used in energy production. Carbon dioxide moves from the tissues to the blood stream, where it is returned via the veins to the right atrium and ultimately to the lungs where it is released into the atmosphere.

GAS TRANSPORT

The red blood cells of the blood are the transportation vehicle for blood gases. Both oxygen and carbon dioxide are moved in this way. Both are carried in solution in blood plasma and combined with hemoglobin.

WORK CAPACITY

Work requires chemical energy to be converted to mechanical energy. This is called metabolism. Metabolism requires oxygen. The volume of oxygen moved by the pulmonary and cardiovascular systems is determined by the persons metabolic needs.

Lung volumes are determined by age, sex and body size. The volume of air breathed by an average person in a minute is six liters. This is a result of an average of 12 breaths per minute and one half liter of air taken in per breath. During vigorous exercise the air moved can be increased significantly. Increases result from an increase in the number of breaths per minute and volume of air taken in with each breath. Trained individuals are capable of increases of up to 17 times that at rest, enabling them to increase the air breathed in a minute to nearly 100 liters.

Normal cardiac output is about 5000 ml. per minute. This is accomplished by two factors, the number of heart beats per minute and the amount of blood pumped per beat (Stroke volume). Trained individuals normally have a lower resting pulse. This is a result of a stronger heart muscle which generates more force thus their stroke volume is greater.

	Cardiac Output		Heart Rate		Stroke Volume
Sedentary	5000 ml	=	70 beats/min	X	71 ml
Trained	5000 ml	=	50 beats/min	X	100 ml

During vigorous exercise both the sedentary and trained person can increase cardiac output as a result of their heart beating more rapidly. They also can increase cardiac output as a result of increases in stroke volume. Trained persons usually have a much greater increase. The sedentary person may have an increased cardiac output up to four times that of resting, while the trained person's increase can be up to seven times greater.

SUMMARY

The cardiovascular and pulmonary systems are responsible for the transportation and circulation of oxygen. Air enters the body and is transported to the lungs. In the lungs oxygen is loaded into the blood stream where it travels to the left atrium. The left atrium pumps the blood to the left ventricle which in turn pumps it to all of the tissues of the body. At the tissue level, oxygen moves from the blood to the tissues where it is used in the production of energy. Carbon dioxide, a by-product of energy production, moves from the tissues to the blood stream. It is carried to the right atrium which pumps it to the right ventricle. The right ventricle pumps this blood to the lungs, where the carbon dioxide moves from the blood to the lungs and is exhaled.

Metabolic needs determine the oxygen needs of the body. The trained individual has a much greater reserve capacity for circulating and transporting oxygen.

WORKSHEET 4-A

Chapter Four—Systems of the Body
Cardiovascular and Pulmonary

Select A or B and record in the appropriate space.

1. The human heart has (A. 2) chambers (B. 4) chambers.   1. _____

2. The upper chambers are called (A. Ventricles) or (B. Atria).   2. _____

3. The bottom chambers are called (A. Atria) or (B. Ventricles).   3. _____

4. The chamber that receives deoxygenated blood is (A. Rt. Atrium) or (B. L. Ventricle).   4. _____

5. The chamber that receives oxygenated blood from the lungs is (A. L. Atrium) or (B. Rt. Ventricle).   5. _____

6. The primary pump of the human heart is (A. Rt. Atrium) or (B. L. Ventricle).   6. _____

7. The chamber that pumps blood to and from the lungs is (A. Rt. Atrium) or (B. Rt. Ventricle).   7. _____

8. The circulatory system that carries oxygenated blood to the cells is (A. Arterial) or (B. Venous).   8. _____

9. The circulatory system that carries deoxygenated blood back to the heart is (A. Arterial) or (B. Venous).   9. _____

10. The blood vessel that has a pulse is (A. Artery) or (B. Vein).   10. _____

11. The blood vessel that has system of one way valves is (A. Artery) or (B. Vein).   11. _____

12. In what blood vessels is the gas exchanged (A. Venule) or (B. Capillary).   12. _____

13. The blood pressure is higher in what blood vessel (A. Artery) or (B. Vein).   13. _____

14. The blood pressure that measures how hard the heart is working is (A. Systolic) or (B. Diastolic).   14. _____

15. The blood pressure that measures the resistance in the blood vessels is (A. Systolic) or (B. Diastolic).   15. _____

16. Normal systolic blood pressure is (A. 210) or (B. 120).   16. _____

17. Normal diastolic blood pressure is (A. 80) or (B. 180).   17. _____

18. The total of all the chemical reactions that occur in the body is called (A. Metabolism) or (B. Catabolism).   18. _____

19. External respiration occurs in the (A. Lungs) or (B. Heart).   19. _____

20. Internal respiration occurs in the (A. Lungs) or (B. Body Cell).   20. _____

21. The arteries that supply the heart with fuel are (A. Coronary) or (B. Brachial).   21. _____

CHAPTER FIVE
Body Composition, Type & Build

One of the most common reasons for beginning an exercise program is the concept of body shaping. Particularly for women, this perceived body shape that is portrayed in the marketing of health and fitness products is a very strong motivator. Outside of a loss of total body weight, it is probably the biggest motivator.

People are led to believe that they are supposed to look like these models, and that if they buy this product or service, they will. At best this is highly unlikely to occur, and most often it becomes a strong disincentive to exercise.

The following will explain the role of body shaping in an exercise/activity program.

The primary reason people have the body shape they do is because of heredity. Heredity's influence determines his/her body type and body build. **BODY BUILD** is heredity's influence on the cross sectional size, width and length of the skeletal system, and **BODY TYPE** is heredity's influence on the amount and distribution of the soft tissue, muscle and fat.

BODY BUILD

In body build, the individual has virtually no control of the skeletal system outside of protecting it from trauma. The long bones in the legs determine the height of the person. The flat bones in the hips and shoulders determine the width of the person. The cross sectional size of the long bones influence the girth of the arms and legs, while the cross sectional size of the flat bones in the hips, shoulders and chest influence the girth of the torso. The body build is essentially the infrastructure of the body shape, and change is beyond the control of the individual.

BODY TYPE

In body type, the individual has limited control because he/she can influence to a certain degree the amount of fat and muscle tissue on the body. Notice that the emphasis is on limited personal control, because he/she cannot make drastic changes that reverse heredity. One can work within the limits of heredity but cannot erase its' effects.

Through proper diet and exercise, one can increase lean tissue while reducing fat tissue, but all within the limitations established by heredity. With this understood, individuals can enjoy the benefits of a prudent life style while enhancing his/her self image, instead of experiencing the frustration of attempting to achieve unrealistic goals.

SOMATOTYPE

In an attempt to classify heredity's influence on body shape, the concept of somatotyping is often used. **Somatotyping** proposes that there are three general categories of body shape, and that the individual is a combination to a certain degree of all three. The degree of influence from each one varies from person to person.

The three categories of somatotyping are:

Ectomorph—Long, long bones, narrow flat bones, low body fat, small muscles, prominent facial features.
Endomorph—Short long bones, broad flat bones, higher body fat, large muscles, rounded facial features.
Mesomorph—Short long bones, broad shoulder flat bones, narrow flat hip bones, low body fat, large muscles, triangular facial features.

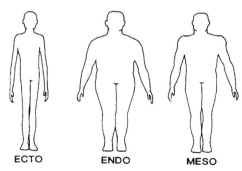

Figure 5-1 Somatotyping

To get an estimate of personal somatotype influence, complete the following:

ECTOMORPH—Record Height _____

Record Percentile Rank of Height _____

Note: To get percentile rank refer to Appendix IV for Males and Appendix V for Females.

Interpretation: If your height is in the higher percentiles, you have a high ectomorphic influence, low percentiles means low influence, etc.

ENDOMORPH—Record six girth scores

Forearm _____ % _____		Waist _____ % _____
Upper Arm _____ % _____		Thigh _____ % _____
Chest _____ % _____		Calf _____ % _____

Note: Use same appendix as above. Interpretation is the same also. The higher the percentile score, the higher the degree of endomorphic influence.

MESOMORPH—Record Body Fat % _____

Record Percentile _____

Note: Use same appendix as above.

Interpretation: Compare the percentile of body fat to the percentile of girth scores. If the body fat is low and the girth is high, the mesomorphic influence is greater. If the reverse is true, high fat, low girth, the influence is low.

BODY COMPOSITION

Total body weight is meaningless. What is important is how much of that total weight is making a positive contribution and how much of is adversely affecting overall well being. This relationship is called **BODY COMPOSITION** and is expressed as a percentage of body fat.

The following chart 5-1 shows that the fat percentage needs to be in an optimal range. In other words, an individual needs a certain amount of fat, but not too much.

CHART 5-1

FAT PERCENTAGES		
	MALES	**FEMALES**
UNDERFAT	0-4	0-12
ACCEPTABLE	5-15	13-23
OVERFAT	16-24	24-32
OBESE	25-+	33-+

As the chart 5-1 implies, the human needs a certain amount of fat because it provides the vital functions of fuel supply, protection, insulation and contouring. The category of acceptable means that the person has enough fat to carry out those aforementioned essential functions. It implies that the current lifestyle of the person is providing an appropriate ratio of food intake to energy output.

Overfat simply means that the person is either eating too much or is underactive, or a combination of both. It implies that the person is producing more fat than is necessary. Obesity is a very serious condition because it has been documented as having many adverse affects on the quality and longevity of life. It requires immediate attention from a licensed health care practitioner.

ESTIMATING BODY FAT

There are a number of ways of estimating body composition, with the three most common methods currently being used are hydrostatic weighing, electrical impedance and skin fold calipers. Of the three, the most common is skin fold measurements due to its inexpense, efficacy and accuracy.

The rationale of skin fold measurements is that the human being prefers to store fat in predetermined locations on the body. The male stores fat in the chest, abdomen and thighs. Females store fat on the triceps, hips and thighs. The skin fold method simply measures the amount of fat at those locations by pinching it using an instrument called a caliper. The data generated from that measurement is then put into a formula and an estimate of the percentage of body fat is made.

SKIN FOLD CALCULATION METHOD

Record the three site scores.

	MALES			**FEMALES**
CHEST	_____	TRICEPS		_____
ABDOMEN	_____	HIPS		_____
THIGH	_____	THIGH		_____
TOTAL	_____	TOTAL		_____

The total is called the Sum of Skinfolds. Males refer to Appendix I, Females refer to Appendix II. Plot your total score in the first column on the left called Sum of Skinfold. Next, go to the appropriate age column and go down that column until age column intersects with the Sum of Skinfolds column. That intersection of the Sum and Age columns is the estimate of body fat.

BODY FAT ESTIMATE _____%.

Name _____ Grade _____

Chapter Five—Body Composition, Body Build and Body Type

Body Composition Chart—Record Personal Data:

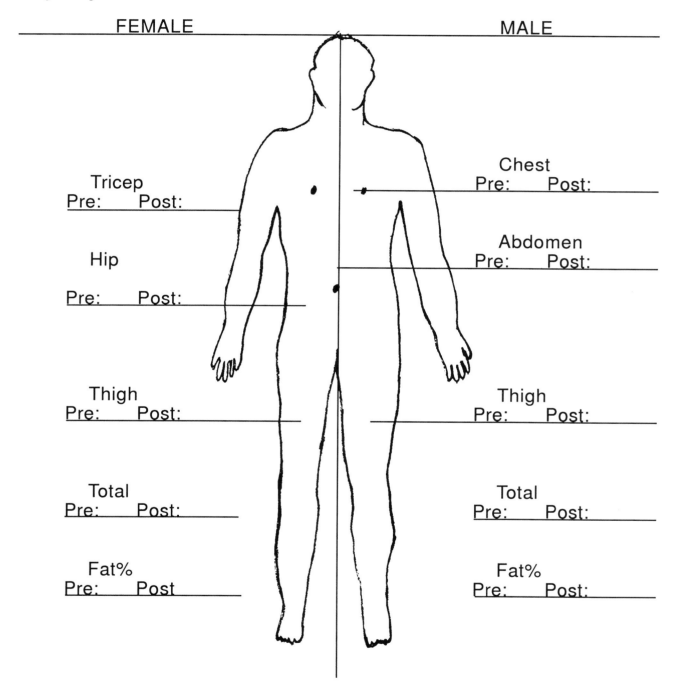

FEMALE   MALE

Tricep
Pre: Post:

Chest
Pre: Post:

Hip

Pre: Post:

Abdomen
Pre: Post:

Thigh
Pre: Post:

Thigh
Pre: Post:

Total
Pre: Post:

Total
Pre: Post:

Fat%
Pre: Post

Fat%
Pre: Post:

Figure 5A-1

Name _____ Grade _____

Chapter Five—Body Composition, Body Build and Body Type

Girth Measurement Chart—Record personal data:

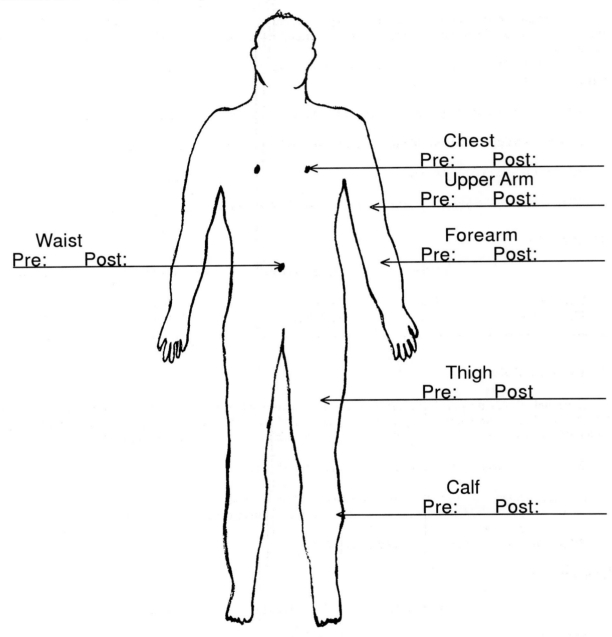

Chest
Pre: Post:

Upper Arm
Pre: Post:

Forearm
Pre: Post:

Waist
Pre: Post:

Thigh
Pre: Post

Calf
Pre: Post:

Figure 5A-2

WORKSHEET 5-C

Chapter Five—Body Composition, Body Build and Body Type

Body Mass Index

Another method of evaluating the height/weight relationship with regard to acceptability is called the *Body Mass Index*. It provides a reference to health related risks resulting from obesity. In general the higher the index the greater the health risk.

It is calculated using the metric system which will require converting height and weight into meters and kilograms respectively. The conversions are as follows:

How to get weight in kilograms? Divide current weight by 2.2 = _____

How to get height in meters? Multiply height in inches by .0254 = _____

And then square that height answer = _____

BMI Formula: Kilograms Wt. Divided by Meters Ht. Squared = _____

Interpretation:

	LEAN	ACCEPTABLE	OVERWEIGHT	OBESE
MALES	< 21.8	21.9-27.2	27.3-30.8	31.9 >
FEMALES	< 21.2	21.3-26.8	26.9-31.3	31.4 >

Waist to Hip Ratio

A method of evaluating girth related to health risks is called the *Waist to Hip Ratio*. It requires two measurements—the waist and hip circumference using either the English or Metric system. It is done in the following manner by wrapping a flexible tape measure snuggly around the body part (do not compress the skin surface.):

Waist measurement—measure the narrowest section of the bare waist while standing. _____

Hip measurement—measure the widest section of the area defined as either the hip, thighs or buttocks while wearing tight fitting clothes and standing. _____

WHR Formula: Waist Girth divided by Hip Girth = _____

Interpretation:

	LOW RISK	AVERAGE RISK	HIGH RISK
MALES	< .90	.91-.95	.96 >
FEMALES	< .80	.81-.85	.86 >

GIRTH MEASUREMENT

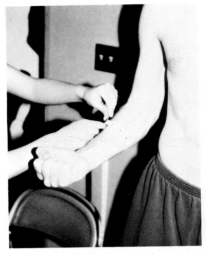

Forearm

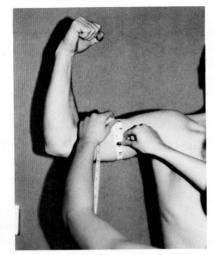

Upper Arm

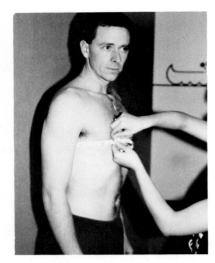

Chest

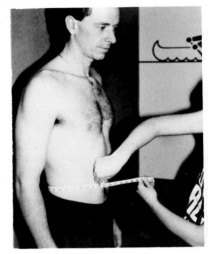

Waist

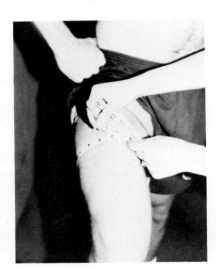

Thigh

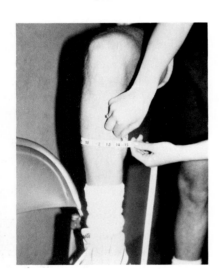

Calf

Figure 5A-3

THREE SITE SKINFOLD MEASUREMENTS

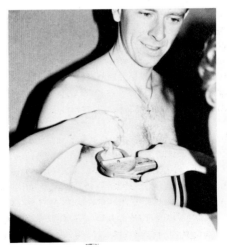

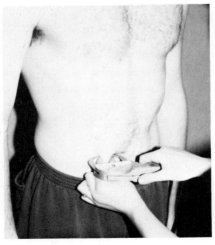

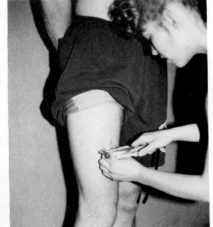

Figure 5A-4

CHAPTER SIX
Basic Nutrition
Fueling the body for Fitness

Of all the factors that have helped shape the fitness surge of the last decade, one area that Americans have been slow to incorporate into their fitness regimes is the concept of healthy, nutritious eating. As Americans, we remain very unaware of the needs of our bodies and how to fuel the body. Countless thousands remain on never ending diets, relying on fast foods and junk foods, and expect that mega-doses of vitamins will keep us healthy and increase our longevity. As our hectic lives keep us hard pressed for time, we look for dietary shortcuts to increase time for other more pressing activities. We need to critically evaluate our nutritional patterns and increase our awareness of food and its value.

The focus of this chapter is to enable you to take a more critical look at your eating patterns and determine if there is room for improvement. If change is necessary, this chapter will lay the foundation for you to become a more educated consumer of food. Other anticipated outcomes will be for you to become better acquainted with reading food labels, to understand the new food pyramid and to understand the best way to lose weight is to eat less (yet nutritious) and increase physical activity.

INTRODUCTION AND REVIEW

When discussing nutrition, we must first develop a basic understanding of the function of food and how the body utilizes what we consume. Simply stated, our bodies are a machine and the foods that we consume provide energy for the engine. If the fuel is of poor quality (junk food, fast food, etc), then the end results over time will also be poor. These results range from weight problems, adult related diabetes, high triglyceride levels, high blood cholesterol and low levels of energy.

When the fuel is of better quality, complex carbohydrates and foods lower in fats, the results are more energy, better weight management, less risk of hypokinetic disease and many more. To understand nutrition, many of you have been raised to understand the 4 Food Groups and their value to the body. Within the last couple of years the focus has changed from the 4 Food Groups to the Food Pyramid (see Figure 6-1).

The food guide pyramid is provided by the United States Department of Agriculture (USDA) and incorporates some material from the original 4 food groups. The changes have been in the increase of complex carbohydrates which are now recognized as being excellent energy sources that are also low in fat. The base of the food pyramid is the bread, cereal, rice and pasta group. It is now recommended that we consume between 6-11 servings every day from this group. The next level of the Food Pyramid is the vegetable group where 3-5 servings are recommended, and the fruit group which suggests 2-4 servings. This is a continuation of increasing the amount of complex carbohydrates that we consume every day.

The next layer of the food pyramid is to eat 2-3 servings from the milk, yogurt, and cheese group. Also at the same level is food from the meat, poultry, fish, dry beans, eggs and nut group. Again the recommendation is to only consume between 2-3 servings from this group daily. At the top of the pyramid is the strong suggestion to use fats, oils and sweets sparingly. The biggest problem that faces many Americans as we try to learn to eat better is that we currently have inverted the pyramid and consume most of our foods from the top of the pyramid and eat less from the fruits, vegetables and grain groups. Now let us further discuss each of these groups.

The foundation of a healthy diet is to increase the amount of complex carbohydrates within our diets. The food from the breads, cereals and grains are the cornerstone of increasing the amount of complex carbohydrates within our diets. In addition, we also increase the amount of fiber that is extremely beneficial to our digestive system. The important nutrients that are provided from the breads, cereals, grains are riboflavin, thiamine, niacin, iron, and protein. Additionally, a good guideline to follow with the purchase or consumption of bread, grains, pasta or cereal is that the darker is better. Whole grain products that have not been bleached during processing provide more fiber and contribute substantially more nutrients than bleached grain products. So whenever possible make the change to whole grain breads and pastas.

Fruits and vegetables are the second most important food group as they are also complex carbohydrates. Unfortunately, many Americans consumption of vegetables is from fast food french fries, and cheese (fat laden) covered vegetables. The important nutrients found within this group are vitamins A & C, riboflavin, and iron. It is important to understand that fruits and vegetables are high in complex carbohydrates, naturally low in fat and are an excellent addition to all healthy diets. Examples of a serving is 1/2 cup of vegetables, an orange, a banana, an apple, or a small salad, with low fat dressing. A medium size apple only has 80 calories, where as a candy bar has roughly 350 calories. A small bag of chips has 180 calories with many of the calories coming from FAT.

Food Guide Pyramid

A Guide to Daily Food Choices

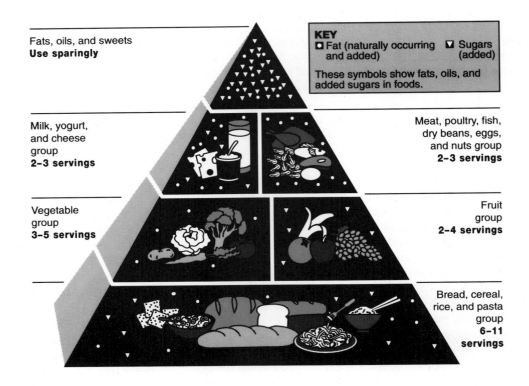

Figure 6-1

Use the Food Guide Pyramid to help you eat better everyday . . . the Dietary Guidelines way. Start with plenty of Breads, Cereals, Rice, and Pasta, Vegetables, and Fruits. Add two to three servings from the Milk group and two to three servings from the Meat group. Each of these food groups provides some, but not all, of the nutrients you need. No one food group is more important than another—for good health you need them all. Go easy on the fats, oils, and sweets, the foods in the small tip of the Pyramid

To order a copy of "The Food Guide Pyramid" booklet, send a $1.00 check or money order made out to the Superintendent of Documents to: Consumer Information Center
Department 159-Y
Pueblo, Colorado 81009
U.S. Department of Agriculture, Human Nutrition Information Service, August 1992, Leaflet No. 572

The foods that are recommended to be a smaller part of our daily diet come from both the dairy and meat groups of the food pyramid. Both of these groups are recommended to consist of no more than 2–3 servings. The primary reason that these foods are not as important to our daily diet is that they tend to be higher in fat content and thus not as healthy. The important nutrients found in the dairy group are calcium, riboflavin, protein, fat and Vitamins A & D. Examples of serving size are 8 ozs. of milk, 1 cup of yogurt, 2 cups of cottage cheese, and 1 cup of ice cream/frozen yogurt. As with the grain group, better choices do exist within the dairy group. Non-fat yogurt, low-fat milk, low-fat cheeses, low-fat ice cream or frozen yogurt are examples of better, healthier choices. It is especially important to try and stay away from processed cheeses.

As consumers you need to learn that although dairy products are important for bone growth and development, it also contributes fat to our diet. Milk is an area that we can make significant changes with our fat consumption and still provide the nutrients our bodies require. Milk is sold in varieties (based on fat content, not white, chocolate, strawberry). Whole milk contains approximately 67% milk fat, 2% milk contains roughly 35% milk fat, 1% milk contains 16% milk fat, and skim milk contains less that 1% milk fat. The recommendation is to make the change to 1% milk, thereby lowering your daily fat intake and still providing the essential milk fat that the body requires.

Additionally, whenever you purchase cottage cheese, yogurt, or many of the cheeses that we consume, look for the lower fat versions that are being prepared to meet consumers demands for better, healthier choices.

> **Outside Project:** Purchase 4— ½ pints of milk; whole, 2% milk, 1% milk and skim milk. Pour each into a glass and mix them with the recommended amount of chocolate mix into each glass. Which milk mixes very well and has very little chocolate that settles to the bottom of the glass? Which milk mixes poorly and has the most chocolate on the bottom? The chocolate mix is adhering to the milk fat, therefore the more milk fat the better it stays mixed.

Within the meat, fish, poultry, nuts and legumes area of the pyramid, the essential ingredients from this food group are protein, iron, niacin, vitamins B-6 and B-12. Serving sizes for this group are a three ounce serving of lean meat, 1 egg (allowing no more than 2 eggs with yolks per week), ½ cup of nuts, seeds or beans.

Here again the choices we make and the quantities that we consume have a direct effect on how the body's systems function. We can reduce the amount of fat we eat by following some simple guidelines. Remove all visible fat before cooking, remove poultry's skin before eating, choose better methods of preparation (cooking over a flame instead of frying, using a wok) use leaner cuts of meat, eat less processed meats like bologna, hot dogs, pepperoni, and reduce the number of times that you have "seconds".

The last area of the pyramid that must be discussed is the area of others (fats, sugars, oils, sweets). Within this area, we find many of the pitfalls that many Americans experience. This group is primarily made up of fat and simple carbohydrates (i.e. refined sugar, butter, margarine, condiments, salt, alcohol, junk food and sweets). These items are often thought of as "empty calories", which contribute high calories with no real nutritional value. By understanding that they are empty calories in terms of key ingredients and high caloric content, we are wise to avoid them or at least significantly reduce our intake. There is no daily recommended servings from this category but less is obviously better.

One aspect when discussing our diet is how often the last group of others is often consumed. The average American consumes over a 100 pounds of refined sugar every year and only roughly 25 to 30 pounds of fruit. If we are to be successful in changing our eating patterns, we must make a concentrated effort to increase the amount of complex carbohydrates we consume and lower the amount of fat and refined sugar. Americans must come to terms with the concept that we are indeed a nation that enjoys fat. We are unfortunately a nation that appears to be addicted to fat and until we understand this, it will take a lot to make positive strides in changing to a more healthy diet.

By incorporating the food pyramid we can start the process of changing to a well balanced healthy diet. The percentages of food in our daily diet is another aspect that can be looked at when discussing a healthy diet. It is recommended that our daily diet consist of 55–60% carbohydrates, 20–30% fat (with no more than 10% being from saturated fat), and 12–15% protein. When examining these percentages it appears odd that fats are the second most necessary ingredient when we keep discussing how unhealthy fat is. What we must consider is that the average American consumes over 40% of their daily calories from fat and yet it is only recommended that the percentage be between 20–30%. Fat is an excellent energy source for the body but as consumption increases more than usage, it becomes stored in the fat cells, which can lead to weight and appearance problems. One of the most significant factors for changing your eating patterns is that by reducing fat and increasing fiber and complex carbohydrates, you significantly decrease the chance of developing heart disease and even death.

In any discussion of a well balanced diet, we must include the 7 Dietary Guidelines developed by the U.S. Department of Agriculture.

1. To eat a variety of foods from the food pyramid.

1. To eat a variety of foods from the food pyramid.
2. To avoid excessive fat, especially saturated fat and cholesterol.
3. To maintain your ideal body weight, based on your frame size, height, weight, and body composition.
4. To increase and consume adequate amounts of complex carbohydrates, starch and fiber.
5. To reduce and avoid too much sugar.
6. To decrease the daily amount of salt.
7. If you drink alcohol, then do so in moderation allowing no more than 1-2 drinks per day.

By including these seven guidelines, we can start to influence and change our dietary habits to a more healthy pattern. Through consumption of the proper servings from the food pyramid we are more likely to consume the 11 key ingredients that our bodies require to function optimally. The 11 key ingredients are carbohydrates, fats, protein, water, thiamin, riboflavin, niacin, iron, calcium and Vitamin A and C. Do they exist in your diet? Are they in the proper amounts?

FURTHER DISCUSSION OF THE 11 KEY INGREDIENTS

Carbohydrates

Carbohydrates are the primary source of energy for the human body and need to comprise 55-60% of our daily diet. There are two types of carbohydrates, complex and simple. Simple carbohydrates are found in refined sugars, sucrose, and are most often found in cookies, candy, soda, honey and cakes. Simple carbohydrates do provide energy for the body but are usually lacking in nutritional value. The guidelines for consumption of simple carbohydrates is that they should not make up more than 10% of our daily calories. In other words a candy bar, a piece of cake or a soda is allowed, but on a very limited basis.

The better source of energy is found within complex carbohydrates such as breads, pasta, cereal, rice, fruits and vegetables. A positive contribution from complex carbohydrates is the increased fiber content added to our diet. There are two types of fiber—insoluble fiber which has been found to lower colon cancer risk and soluble fiber which has been found to decrease blood cholesterol levels.

Carbohydrates are important for us within any discussion of fitness, as they are the primary energy source for the 600 muscles in the body. Carbohydrates are readily broken down into glycogen which can be stored in the muscles. As you examine your eating patterns, you may find that the carbohydrate levels in your diet are lacking and need to be increased. The increase consumption will provide greater energy for your day to day activities and less likelihood of relying on snack/junk foods.

Fats

Much of the literature on nutrition has identified fat as a major health risk for Americans. The problem lies not with fat per se, but rather with the types and amounts that are consumed. Remember that it is recommended that only 20-30% of our daily calories come from fats. The problem is that we average over 40-45% in our daily diet and most of this fat comes from saturated (bad) fats.

Fats (triglycerides) are an excellent energy source and also serve to insulate and protect the internal organs. Triglycerides are found in two types: saturated and unsaturated. Saturated fats come primarily from animal sources (i.e. meats, butter, milk, and also found in coconut and palm oils). Saturated fats are easily identifiable as they are usually solid at room temperature. Saturated fats should never comprise more than 10% of our daily caloric intake.

The other type of fats are known as unsaturated and are found in plant and fish (Omega 3 Fatty Acids). The better choices of unsaturated fat are called monounsaturated fats and include olive, peanut, and canola oil. The other type of good fats are identified as polyunsaturated fats and include corn, safflower and vegetable oils.

Through consumption of a high saturated fat diet, we increase the levels of LDL (commonly referred to as bad cholesterol) and increase the risk of heart disease and cancer. With better food choices, we can increase the HDL (good cholesterol) and thereby reduce the chance of clogging our arteries with fat. Exercise is another method of increasing the HDL and thereby increasing our overall fitness.

Protein

Protein is thought of as the body building and repair material. The body is unable to store protein, therefore it must be consumed every day. Protein is vital to every cell in the body. The problem arises that for many the consumption of protein is greater than the recommended allowance of 12-15%. The consumption of proteins is often associated with an increased addition of fat to our caloric intake.

Protein is identified as amino acids, and 22 amino acids have been identified as necessary for the body. The body is unable to make 9 of these amino acids known as the essential aminos, and therefore must be consumed every day through protein consumption.

There is a large misconception in the field of fitness surrounding protein. Many believe that protein is so important in building muscles, that we should consume more than the recommended amount. This thinking is totally unfounded and has no scientific validity. Our daily consumption should stay within the recommended guidelines. Taking supplements in forms of protein powders and extra servings of meat will most likely lead to weight problems and expensive urine. To develop more muscle on your body, we don't require more protein. What is necessary is more strength resistive exercise using primarily free weights.

Vitamins, Minerals, Water

Vitamins are organic substances that are found in a variety of different foods. Their primary function is to act as regulators of the body (unleashing the energy of carbohydrates, fats and proteins). Through consumption of a well balanced diet, supplementary vitamins are not warranted and are wasteful. Let's examine the 5 vitamins, discuss good food sources for each and identify the functions they serve in the body.

Vitamin A is found in fortified milk, liver, carrots, tomatoes and is helpful with vision, bone growth and repair, as well as its importance to the skin.

Vitamin C is found in all citrus fruits, tomatoes and is important in the healing of wounds. It is also useful in the maintenance of the body's connective tissue and is extremely important for maintaining healthy teeth.

Vitamin Bl (thiamine) is commonly found in the whole grains and lean cuts of meats. Thiamine is helpful in the release of energy from carbohydrates as well as its importance for a healthy heart and nervous system.

Vitamin B2 (riboflavin) is found in nuts, liver and dairy products. Riboflavin as with all of the B complex vitamins help with the release of energy from carbohydrates.

Vitamin B3 (niacin) is also found in nuts, liver, and dairy products. It is important for normal functioning of skin and the digestive system.

There are two minerals that are included within on the 11 key ingredients, they are calcium and iron. Minerals are inorganic substances that are essential to a variety of functions, from digestion to bone formation.

Calcium is essential to the formation of bone and teeth, muscular contraction and blood clotting. Good sources of calcium are dairy products, leafy green vegetables and shellfish.The recommended daily allowance is 800 milligrams for adults and 1200 milligrams for children and pregnant women. The main negative outcome from a calcium deficient diet is osteoporosis, which is reduced bone density and is fairly common with post-menopausal women.

Iron is found in liver, red meats, egg yolks, dried fruits, peas, beans, and green leafy vegetables. Iron is essential to the health of hemoglobin, the body's oxygen supplier. Without oxygen being transported to the body, the cells function poorly and eventually cell death occurs. It is recommended that we consume 10 milligrams every day, except that pregnant women need to increase their consumption to 15 milligrams every day.

It is important to keep in mind that through a well balanced diet, the recommended allowances of vitamins and minerals can be met and supplementation is not necessary. So instead of spending your money on commercial vitamins, invest it in selecting good healthy choices at the grocery store.

The last essential ingredient is water. Each and every day it is highly recommended that we consume 8 glasses of water. Water is extremely important as the body is primarily comprised of water and water acts as a flushing or cleansing agent of the body. An easy test to determine if you are replenishing water for the body is through the color and smell of the urine. If the color is dark yellow and of strong odor, then we need to increase our intake of water. Within the discussion of water intake, glasses of soda, coffee, tea and juice are not to be included.

That is a quick review of essential ingredients that the body requires to stay healthy, active and full of energy. It cannot be stated strongly enough that if you have a well balanced diet with the proper number of servings as suggested within the food pyramid, you will be healthier and decrease the risks of disease associated with poor eating habits.

Salt

Salt is commonly found as table salt, but it is also found in countless thousands of processed foods that we consume every day. Often we don't view processed foods as high in salt and fats, but they can be the downfall of many healthy diets. Salt can be listed under a variety of names: baking powder, garlic salt, MSG, onion salt, sodium chloride or nitrate and soy sauce. Because salt is listed under so many names, removing salt from the diet is a difficult process. Removing salt shakers from our kitchen tables and cooking stations is a good first step, but it is not enough. We must become educated consumers who are wary of many processed foods. Other ways are to incorporate different herbs and spices for flavor enhancement when cooking.

Sodium functions to regulate the water balance in the body and is also involved in controlling blood pressure. The recommended daily allowance varies, but it is usually between 1000-2000 milligrams. Unfortunately, the average American consumes two to three times that amount.

Sugar

The question is often posed as to how harmful is sugar. Much of the research indicates that sugar is not as much of a problem as fat consumption is. Yet sugar can be harmful because it delivers only empty calories that increase the likelihood of causing a positive caloric balance..

Sugar is similar to sodium in that it is packaged under a variety of names, and as consumers we must be informed and be aware of the different names. Sugar is listed as brown sugar, honey, corn syrup, corn sweetener, dextrose, glucose, maltose, sucrose and cane sugar. The most important concept regarding sugar is that sugar (simple carbohydrates) are totally empty calories. If you are watching your caloric intake, then sugar is often seen as a problem area. Otherwise, the recommendation is that no more than 10% of our daily caloric intake should come from the simple carbohydrates (refined sugar).

Starting to Become an Informed Consumer

There are countless ways to become a more health conscious consumer of food. First and foremost is to truly believe that eating healthy is important to you and making a commitment to improve the foods that you provide your body.

Probably, the most significant manner to improve your eating habits is to learn how to read labels and analyze the foods that we are eating. As we read labels, we begin by running through the list of ingredients, which are listed from the most to the least within that food. We also are looking for hidden sugars, utilizing the different names previously addressed. It is also important to look for the word hydrogenated added to any oils, as this process changes a healthy fat into an unhealthy fat.

The next step in reading labels is to determine what percentage of the calories come from what food group. There is a simple rule used to calculate where the calories come from in all food stuffs. The rule is known as the 4-4-9 rule. For each gram of carbohydrate and protein listed in the food there are 4 calories per gram. So if a food has 14 grams of carbohydrates listed then you would multiply 14 X 4 to come up with 56 calories from carbohydrates. For every gram of fat per serving in the food, you would multiply the number of grams by 9 to calculate the total number of calories from fat.

You then may determine the percentages of food by dividing the number of calories of either fat, protein or carbohydrates by the total calories per serving.

Eating Disorders

Unfortunately, any discussion regarding increased awareness of nutrition must also include at least the introduction of eating disorders. In this day and age, many people are trying to achieve the perfect body with unreasonable expectations and outcomes. The first question is what is the perfect body? The answer is obvious, there is no such thing as the perfect body. Yes, there are many examples of what may be considered the perfect body, but research indicates that many variables affect our bodies. These variables range from body type, hereditary, Basal Metabolic Rate, eating behavior, and exercise intensity.

Eating disorders are an outcome of our culture's emphasis on thinness and are both medical and psychiatric disorders that affect many women and some men. The eating disorders we will briefly discuss are Anorexia Nervosa and Bulimia Nervosa.

Anorexia Nervosa—Persons suffering from this illness are usually slightly overweight and start dieting to loose the weight. They starve themselves and increase the amount of exercise they are doing. As they start to loose the weight, they distort their perceptions of self and become obsessed with thinness. This continues as they continue to view themselves as fat and continue the starvation manner. Often times this obsession with thinness leads to chemical imbalances that can lead to organ damage and in some cases death. Any person suffering with anorexia needs counseling and will probably require hospitalization.

Bulimia Nervosa—Persons suffering from this illness often have an intense fear of gaining weight and becoming fat. Bulimics tend to binge and purge as the manner of controlling their weight. They binge by eating many calories and then feel guilty and try to remove the calories from their system. Initially, they rely on making themselves vomit but as they become more involved they start using laxatives and diuretics. Serious side effects are kidney failure and heart arrythmias. As with anorexics, bulimics will require counseling to deal with the poor self image and any other underlying causes.

Final Thoughts

The intention of this chapter was to provide a quick cook's tour of the basics regarding a healthy, well balanced diet. It was a quick overview that hopefully will interest the reader to further pursue more on the topic of good nutrition. By implementing the food pyramid, the 7 rules of good nutrition and looking at what we eat, we are indeed on the way to a better, healthier lifestyle.

Remember that the "complete package" when discussing fitness is not only the amount of activity that we incorporate into our lifestyles, but also the fuel and energy we provide through our eating patterns. Good Luck as you begin your journey to a healthier lifestyle, both through good nutrition and increased activity.

WORKSHEET 6-A

Chapter Six—Examining A Day's Eating Pattern

The focus of this lab is to record all the foods eaten in one day. You will also be asked to identify the calories from each food for that day. At the end of the day, you are to review the Food Pyramid and determine if you met the suggested foods for that day. The last question is do you consider this day to be a healthy diet or one that needs improvement.

Items Eaten	Time of Day	Approximate Calories	Food Group

Do you consider your diet to be a healthy diet?   YES   NO

What suggestions would you make to improve your diet, to make it more healthy? List as many as you feel are reasonable for you.

_____

_____

_____

_____

_____

_____

_____

_____

_____

_____

_____

WORKSHEET 6-B

Chapter Six—Examining A Day's Eating Pattern

Identify Food Group

Put the letter of the food group next to the food listed. If the food is a combination put both, refer to Appendix III.

A—Fat	**B—Carbohydrate**	**C—Protein**

FOOD	GROUP	FOOD	GROUP
1. Oils	1. _____	36. Pizza Cheese	36. _____
2. Milk	2. _____	37. Popcorn	37. _____
3. Vegetables	3. _____	38. Potato Chips	38. _____
4. Meat	4. _____	39. French Fries	39. _____
5. Poultry	5. _____	40. Pretzels	40. _____
6. Fish	6. _____	41. Cola	41. _____
7. Eggs	7. _____	42. Spaghetti Sauce	42. _____
8. Nuts	8. _____	43. Taco Bell Taco	43. _____
9. Fruits	9. _____	44. Tortilla Chips	44. _____
10. Bread	10. _____	45. Tuna/water	45. _____
11. Cereal	11. _____	46. Whopper	46. _____
12. Rice	12. _____	47. Whopper w/Cheese	47. _____
13. Pasta	13. _____	48. Wine	48. _____
14. Cheese	14. _____	49. Whiskey	49. _____
15. Yogurt	15. _____	50. Tea	50. _____
16. Bagel	16. _____		
17. Beer	17. _____		
18. Brownies	18. _____		
19. Butter	19. _____		
20. Taco Bell Burrito	20. _____		
21. McDs Cheeseburger	21. _____		
22. Chicken McNuggets	22. _____		
23. Coffee	23. _____		
24. Corn Chips	24. _____		
25. Plain Donut	25. _____		
26. Egg McMuffin	26. _____		
27. Hot Dog	27. _____		
28. Big Mac	28. _____		
29. Hot Dog Roll	29. _____		
30. Ice Cream—Vanilla	30. _____		
31. M & C	31. _____		
32. Margarine	32. _____		
33. Chocolate Shake	33. _____		
34. Peanut Butter	34. _____		
35. PB & J Sandwich	35. _____		

CHAPTER SEVEN
Fat Loss—Weight Loss

In Chapter Five the point was made that body shaping was a powerful motivator for people to begin an exercise program. Another equally strong motivator for exercise is to lose total body weight. People perceive exercise as the magic formula needed for them to reach a perceived goal of weight loss.

This process of weight loss and gain is unfortunately not quite that simple. Yes, exercise will help, but it is only part of the formula—not the entire formula. It is the intent of this chapter to clarify the scientific fact specific to these processes.

In most cases people make an incorrect basic assumption—They say they want to lose weight, when in fact what they really want is to lose fat. Weight and fat loss are two completely different processes. Yes, they are related and impact one another, but they are not one in the same.

Total body weight needs to be addressed first. There are three basic components of **total body weight: water weight, lean tissue weight** and **fat tissue weight.** Changes in any one of them will obviously affect the overall total.

WATER WEIGHT

Water comprises about half of the total body weight. Therefore it is essential that the role of water in the fat/weight loss process be understood. Water weight fluctuates on a daily basis because water volume fluctuates on a daily basis. Water is lost through elimination, expiration and perspiration at a rate of about 2 1/2 quarts per day (4-5 lbs.). If that volume is not replaced through rehydration via food and liquid intake, there would be a net loss of body weight on that given day. However, if rehydration was adequate, water weight would remain the same. If too much liquid was retained, as in the female menstrual cycle, there would be a net weight gain.

The most important thing to remember is that in this water weight fluctuation, no lean or fat tissue was gained or lost. There was only a change in water volume and that is very transient.

Programs that purport to offer the consumer rapid weight loss are simply plying on this de/rehydration process. Any body weight lost through dehydration will be rapidly replaced once the rehydration process begins via the diet.

Water is an absolutely essential component of the well balanced diet and should never be restricted. All vital functions of the body are dependent upon adequate water supplies.

LEAN TISSUE

Lean tissue is gained through the normal growth and development process of the human from childhood to adulthood. Once maturation has occurred, lean tissue increase ceases. If further development of lean tissue is desired, then a program of resistance training along with proper diet is required.

The resistance (weight) training is necessary to create the overload on the tissue, which then stimulates the tissue to increase its' protein content. The effect is that the tissue becomes more dense with protein, adding to the total weight of the particular tissue. This increase in protein content is then reflected as an increase in total body weight and is called **hypertrophy.**

(This process will be presented at length in a later chapter.)

The reverse of this process is called **atrophy**, in which lean tissue is lost through a loss of protein content. It occurs as a result of disuse of that tissue. A good example is a person who may have had an arm or leg immobilized by a cast as a result of some trauma. While in the cast, the underlying tissue, bone and muscle, was not used and lost protein content. When the cast was removed there was a noticeable difference in the cross sectional size of the immobilized arm compared to the other arm. This obvious loss of lean tissue would be reflected in a reduction of total body weight.

In summary, lean tissue is generated through the stimulus of prudent physical stress on the tissue. Lean tissue is lost through disuse or the removal of physical stress.

FAT TISSUE

A Calorie is a unit of measurement, which identifies the amount of heat generated in energy consumption and energy output. Everything we eat has an energy equivalent, which is referred to as its caloric value. On the other hand, everything we do to stay alive has an energy cost. The key to controlling fat is to balance the number of calories consumed with the number of calories burned in maintaining the current lifestyle.

When a person eats more calories in a day than he/she burns, a positive caloric balance is realized and those extra calories are stored as fat. If that positive caloric balance accumulates to a total of 3,500, a pound of fat would be gained. An example would be a person who has a positive caloric balance of 100 calories a day for 35 consecutive days. That person would then have gained a pound of fat over that time. So any combination of positive caloric balances equalling 3500 will result in a fat gain.

In the reverse, a negative caloric balance equalling 3500 would result in a loss of a pound of stored fat. Generating negative caloric balances requires the body to use stored fat to meet its daily energy requirements.

The key point to remember is that 3500 is a very large number and not easily reached over short periods of time. Therefore, in reality fat is not gained quickly nor can it be lost quickly. Fat is gained as a result of generating small positive caloric balances over long periods of time. And to lose it properly, that same process should be reversed. That is, generate small, continuous negative caloric balances over long periods of time. In this manner, the lifestyle change necessary to achieve the fat loss will evolve and be more manageable. To attempt to make drastic short term gains is unsustainable.

ROLE OF EXERCISE

Exercise has an energy cost just like any other human activity and can therefore be used to help generate negative caloric balances. But while helping to generate negative caloric balances, exercise can also help to maintain or even generate more lean tissue while isolating fat loss. Studies have shown that weight reduction programs incorporating exercise result in a loss of stored fat only and not lean tissue.

Lean tissue is dense and has an anatomical shape. Fat tissue is not very dense and its shape is more determined by location and gravity than anything else. Per unit of weight, fat has more volume and therefore takes up more space.

CALORIC DEPRIVATION

The least desirable of all weight loss programs is caloric deprivation. Studies have shown that restricting calories without increasing activity or exercise, results in a loss of lean as well as fat tissue. For every pound of weight loss generated by caloric deprivation, half comes from lean tissue (atrophy) and half from fat tissue. The end result is that the person may accomplish weight reduction, but he/she will not contribute much to body shaping. He/she will weigh less but be the same body shape.

Caloric deprivation is also subject to the basal metabolic rate (BMR) adjustment. The BMR is the rate at which the body produces and consumes energy. When the BMR is high, large amounts of energy are used as is the case of exercise or heavy physical labor. However the opposite is true when the body is at rest or when calories are restricted. What happens is that the brain senses a restriction in caloric intake and automatically begins to reduce energy consumption by lowering the BMR as a protective mechanism.

This is why caloric deprivation programs experience early success followed by plateaus. Initially the caloric deprivation generates negative caloric balances resulting in weight loss. However this does not last. The BMR adjusts downward and results in a plateau where no more weight is lost because there are no more negative caloric balances.

If further weight loss is desired, then the person must further reduce intake to achieve negative caloric balances. And then soon after, the BMR again adjusts downward and the same scenario repeats itself.

The caloric deprivation cycle is generally completed when the dieter reaches a level of caloric intake that is so low that it is not sustainable any longer, and he/she begins eating a normal diet. However because the BMR has been driven down so low, this return to normal eating (Approx. 2000 cal./day Females and 3000 cal./day Males) creates huge positive caloric balances and a rapid regaining of the lost weight.

What's worse is that the gained weight will be mostly fat. The net result of this caloric deprivation cycle is that the dieter ends up weighing the same or more but with a much higher fat percentage that when he/she started.

RECOMMENDATIONS

Chart 7-1

Foodstuffs Cal/Gram and % of Diet		
	Cal/Gram	% Diet
Carbohydrate	4.1	60-65
Protein	4.1	15-20
Fat	9.3	25-30

- Limit Fat Intake—Fat is very high in calories and does not generate a lot of volume.
- Eat mostly complex Carbohydrates—Fruits, vegetables, cereals and grains. Provides volume plus nutrition.
- Limit the use of empty calories—sauces, gravies, meat juices, dressings. Empty fat calories.
- Don't skip meals—overeating results.
- Limit processed foods—generally high in calories and salt while low in nutritional content.
- Don't delete foods you like even if high in calories—limit the intake.
- Drink plenty of water—no calories, essential nutritional component.
- Eat smaller amounts more often—easier to digest, avoids hunger pangs and energy sags.
- Eat more calories early in day—better chance to burn them than store them.
- Make changes gradually—evolution is less traumatic and more sustainable that revolution.

WORKSHEET 7-A

Chapter Seven—Caloric Balance Sheet

The purpose of the caloric balance sheet is to estimate whether the person's current lifestyle is generating positive or negative caloric balances.

It first consists of identifying the total energy intake in one given day. This is done by listing the foods consumed in a representative day and assigning a caloric value to them. This is then totalled to get the number of calories consumed in one day.

The next step is to list the activities of the person during this same day and determine the energy costs of those activities. These are also totalled.

The two totals, energy intake and energy output, are then compared to determine if the person is generating positive caloric balances and storing fat, or negative caloric balances and burning stored fat.

Instructions—Caloric Balance Sheet

ENERGY INPUT—List the foods eaten in a normal day in the column under "Food" on the "Energy Input" side of the Balance Sheet. Refer to APPENDIX III—NUTRITIVE VALUE OF SELECTED FOODS to get the caloric value of those individual foods, which is listed in column 3—"Cal." Write down the caloric value for each individual food on the list under the column "Caloric Input" on the line next to the food and then total all of them at the bottom.

> **Example:**
> Apple—80

ENERGY COSTS—List all of the activities for a normal 24 hour period under the column "Activity" on the "Energy Costs" side of the balance sheet. Refer to APPENDIX II, ENERGY COST OF ACTIVITY to get the caloric value of the activities. Calculate the energy cost of each activity by multiplying the caloric cost by the number of minutes the activity was done and then multiplying that number by the persons body weight. List that number on the line next to the activity under the "Caloric Costs" column. Total that column to get the total energy costs of one day.

> **Example:**
> Sleeping—   .0066
>   x 420 (7 hrs. Sleep - 60 min. x 7 =420 min.)
>   2.77
>   x 160 body weight of the person
>   443.5 Calories burned while sleeping.
>
> Sleeping—443.5
> Eating—
> Walking—

Compare the two "TOTAL" lines. If the Energy Input Column is higher than the Energy Costs Column, then the person is eating more than he/she is burning off and is storing fat. If the reverse is true, he/she is burning off more than is being eaten and stored fat is being reduced.

WORKSHEET 7–A

Chapter Seven—Fat Loss—Weight Loss

CALORIC BALANCE SHEET

Instructions: Refer to Appendix II for Energy costs of Activities and Appendix III for Caloric Food Content.

Energy Costs		**Energy Input**	
Activity	Caloric Cost	Food	Caloric Input
1._____	_____	1._____	_____
2._____	_____	2._____	_____
3._____	_____	3._____	_____
4._____	_____	4._____	_____
5._____	_____	5._____	_____
6._____	_____	6._____	_____
7._____	_____	7._____	_____
8._____	_____	8._____	_____
9._____	_____	9._____	_____
10._____	_____	10._____	_____
11._____	_____	11._____	_____
12._____	_____	12._____	_____
TOTAL	_____		_____

Total Plus/Minus_____

CHAPTER EIGHT
Myths and Fallacies

Answer the following questions based on current knowledge.

True/False

1. A person can target a certain body part for size reduction.
2. To be beneficial, exercise must hurt.
3. Benefits gained from exercise are permanent.
4. Muscle turns to fat when not used.
5. Males are stronger than females biologically.
6. Seniors citizens should not exercise.
7. Prepubescent children should not exercise.
8. If women exercise with weights, they will end up looking like a guy.
9. Women cannot improve their strength lifting weights.
10. Dietary supplements are safe and effective.

1. _____
2. _____
3. _____
4. _____
5. _____
6. _____
7. _____
8. _____
9. _____
10. _____

If you answered true/yes to any of the above questions, your current knowledge about the benefits and effects of exercise is inaccurate.

The following information is intended to present the current scientific fact specific to exercise in the hopes of dispelling many of the myths and fallacies associated with it.

SPOT REDUCING

There is no such thing as spot reducing, regardless of what cable TV commercials say. There is simply no scientific data to support this concept. Proponents of this misbelief state that they can design a program, or they recommend a piece of equipment that will isolate a body part and change (reduce) its size. Women's thighs and men's abdominals are popular targets.

The fact is that size (fat) reduction is a process of generating negative caloric balances that was previously addressed in Chapter Seven. Exercise by itself will help burn calories but not site specific ones.

Exercising the site specific muscles will improve their overall performance but will not by itself reduce the cross sectional size. Also it must be remembered that heredity plays a large part in cross sectional size. What may be interpreted as too large or fat, may in fact be perfectly normal for that particular person because of the inherited body type.

Fat will come off first where it went on last, and there is no willful control of this process.

The best exercise program to be used for generating negative caloric balances is large muscle repetitive endurance types such as walking, aerobic dance, cross country skiing, etc. These forms of exercise offer the person the best method of a continuously higher caloric burn.

NO PAIN NO GAIN

Pain is a form of communication. It is the body telling the person something is wrong. Therefore it is prudent to pay attention to what the body is trying to say.

It is true that the body has to be stressed to improve physically. If an exercise program does not stress the body physically, then little if any improvements can be expected.

However, exercise does not and should not have to painful to be effective.

The key to prudent exercise is to reach a training range that is both safe and effective. How to do this is addressed in another chapter dealing with exercise prescriptions. The most important thing to remember is that if an exercise is causing pain, it is not appropriate and should be stopped. Ignoring pain can lead to acute as well as chronic type overuse injuries. Neither one is acceptable in a prudent exercise program.

HYPERTROPHY

Hypertrophy is an increase in cross sectional size of a body part. It occurs in two ways. The first is called **transient hypertrophy** and results from a fluid shift to the working muscles. (See Chart 8-1) And the second is called **durable hypertrophy** and results from protein being added to the muscle cells.

CHART 8-1

MUSCLE BLOOD FLOW PERCENTAGES			
AT REST	LIGHT EXERCISE	MODERATE EXERCISE	HEAVY EXERCISE
20%	47%	71%	88%

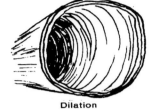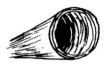

Dilation   Constriction

Figure 8-1 Blood Vessels: Dilation and Constriction

Transient hypertrophy lasts only as long as the exercise bout lasts. It is called "pumping up" and is simply an engorgement of fluid to a working muscle. It is a physiological adaption to work being done by that muscle. The working muscle needs more fuel and the body delivers it via an increase in fluid to the muscle.

Durable hypertrophy occurs when the muscle adds protein content as a result of physical stress being placed on it. It most often results from some form of weight or resistant training that creates an overload on the muscle. The muscle responds to the stress by adding protein content to the individual fibers which then contributes to an overall increase in cross sectional size.

As long as the weight training program continues, the size will be maintained. However, if the person stops weight training, the size gains created by the weight training will be reversed.

The person will then return to his/her normal cross sectional size as determined by the his/her inherited body type. The important point to remember is that what is permanent is what the person got through heredity. Any change that occurs as a result of an exercise program will last only as long as the exercise program that created the change lasts. Hence the word durable is used not permanent.

Sex and body types will affect the durable hypertrophy process. Females with an estrogen dominance will not respond as much as males with a testosterone dominance. Therefore females are unlikely to achieve large cross sectional size gains.

Also, mesomorphs and endormorphs are more likely to see greater hypertrophy than ectomorphs.

MUSCLE TURNS TO FAT

Muscle is muscle. Fat is fat. They are two completely different types of tissue, and the processes for gaining or losing each are completely different also.

Muscle increases in size in response to overload training by adding protein to the individual fibers. The degree of increase is specific to the person's sex, body type and training regimen. Muscle loses size through disuse when protein content is lost.

Fat content increases when life styles generate positive caloric balances of 3500 or more. Fat is lost when life styles generate negative caloric balances of 3500 or more.

The misconception of muscle turning to fat probably comes from the fact that when people stop exercising, they have a tendency to gain weight/fat. They didn't adjust their caloric intake downward to reflect the new less active lifestyle. This then resulted in large positive caloric balances and the creation of stored fat. This in combination with a loss of lean tissue from disuse gives the impression that the muscle they had now turned into fat. When in fact, the two processes are very different although they may have occurred simultaneously.

The important lesson to be learned is that when the lifestyle activity levels change, there must be comparable change in caloric intake. If the lifestyle is very active with high energy costs, such as an in season athlete, more calories are needed in the daily diet to meet these needs. If on the other hand, the lifestyle becomes more sedentary with lower energy costs, such as an out of season athlete, fewer calories are needed in the daily diet.

Lastly, the only way of maintaining or increasing muscle content is through the physical stress of exercise.

MUSCULAR STRENGTH—MALE VS. FEMALE

Who is stronger, the male or the female? With regard to the sum total of all the strength potential in the body, which is called absolute strength, the male is stronger.

Why? The male is stronger because the average male is bigger than the average female. The ability to apply force is subject to the laws of physics. The average male has a distinct leverage advantage because he has longer levers, and more lean, total mass to apply to those levers.

The average male is 5'10" tall, weighs 175 lbs. and has 15% body fat. The average female is 5'4", weighs 130 lbs. and has 23% body fat. The advantage in strength is simply mechanical in nature. Skeletal muscle does not discriminate sexually. It doesn't know whether it is male or female.

Neutralizing the mechanical advantage results in no inherent advantage for one sex over the other.

EXERCISE AND THE SENIOR

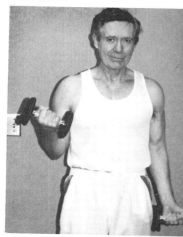

There is no time limit on receiving the benefits from prudent exercise and activity. One is never too old to derive some benefits from a personalized exercise program.

Aging is a relentless process that gradually reduces the functioning level of the human. Physically, the human body becomes less dense through the loss of cells that are not replaced.

Although we cannot stop the aging clock, we can slow the process down. Research has shown that the BMR (the total metabolic activity of the body) is reduced at a rate of 3% per decade after maturation. However, research has also shown that a vigorous and regular activity and/or exercise program can slow this loss to 1% per decade.

So yes, we are going to get old and lose physical capabilities, but we have significant control over the rate of the loss. We can get old quickly, or we can get old slowly. It's essentially up to the individual. The person has the control to retain a higher level of quality of life for longer periods of time through the prudent use of exercise and activity. A sedentary lifestyle simply accelerates the aging process.

EXERCISE AND THE CHILDREN

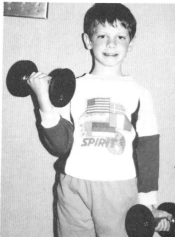

Can prepubescent children benefit from formal exercise programs? It was once thought they could not because hormone levels were inadequate, and that exercise could not increase strength beyond the normal growth curve. This perception has been proven false. Formal exercise for immature children can expedite strength gains above the normal growth curve.

If this is true, then what types of programs are most appropriate? The answer is a personalized, strictly supervised and well planned programs directed by knowledgeable professionals. Children are a very vulnerable group due to the immaturity factor so exercise programs must be strictly controlled.

Outside of formal training programs, informal, spontaneous and self initiated play is by far the best form of activity for the immature child.

WOMEN AND EXERCISE

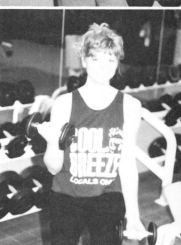

In the past, women were screened out of formal training programs either by themselves or by others in authority. The biggest reason given was that they would end up "looking like a guy", specifically increases in muscle definition and hypertrophy.

Fortunately as it is now known, this is simply not true. Women can get all of the benefits that formal training has to offer without ending up with unwanted definition and size gains.

On average, women have approximately 7% more body fat than males. This accounts for the contouring of the surface anatomy of female and makes muscle definition (prominent skeletal musculature) highly unlikely. Females would have to get to dangerously low levels of body fat before definition would appear. It would not happen by accident and most certainly would represent a health risk for the women. A certain level of body fat is necessary (aprrox. 11% for females) in order for the body to carry on its vital functions. Without adequate levels of this tissue, overall health will suffer. Normal training programs will not reduce body fat levels to the point where definition would occur.

The second concern of females is the issue of hypertrophy. Here again like anatomical surface definition, hypertrophy is not likely to occur because females have a dominance of the sex hormone estrogen, which doesn't appear to be related to increases in skeletal muscle size. The males have a dominant sex hormone called testosterone that is related to hypertrophy of skeletal muscle. So with naturally higher levels of estrogen and naturally lower levels of testosterone, it would be very difficult for the female to achieve skeletal muscle hypertrophy.

In summary, females can get all of the benefits of formal, aggressive training programs without the unwanted outcomes of definition and hypertrophy.

SUPPLEMENTS

The use of dietary supplements without an identified deficiency is essentially a form of self medication. The common scenario is that an individual perceives a need for a vitamin, mineral or foodstuff supplement. This results from word of mouth or other forms of marketing about the benefits of a certain supplement. And then without any confirmation of the need from a reliable and valid source, the person purchases this over the counter product and begins taking it.

At best, it will be just a waste of money. At worst it could result in some form of adverse reaction that can at times be dangerous.

There is no unequivocal scientific evidence in existence that proves that supplements work. The single most important supplement is a balanced, nutritional diet. If a person has a proper diet that meets the needs of the body, no supplements are necessary.

If the person feels that his/her diet is inadequate, the deficiencies should be identified and then addressed directly with the proper supplements. But to assume a deficiency and guess at what it might be is not very prudent.

Different people have different lifestyles with varying degrees of stress contained within them. It is reasonable to assume that dietary deficiencies can exist. But it is the prudent person, who when suspecting a deficiency, will take the necessary steps to determine if there is in fact a deficiency and identify specifically what it is. Then the correct supplement can be utilized to address a confirmed need.

Only in this situation can the person be confident that his/her needs are being met in a safe and effective manner. Any other use of supplements is at best a reckless endeavor that is expensive and can also be harmful. It can actually hurt the person more that it can help them.

WORKSHEET 8-A

Chapter Eight—Myths and Fallacies

True/False

1. There is no such thing as spot reducing.
2. There is scientific support for spot reducing.
3. Females store fat on the upper arms, thighs and hips.
4. Males store fat in the abdomen and buttocks.
5. Fat comes off first where it went on last.
6. Aerobic type activities are best for fat loss.
7. Exercise must hurt to be effective.
8. Pain is form of communication.
9. Ignoring pain can be dangerous.
10. It is not necessary to stress the body physically to improve fitness levels.
11. Exercise does not increase blood flow to working muscles.
12. Pumping up achieves a permanent size gain.
13. Pumping up simply means engorging a working muscle with blood.
14. Permanent size gains are achieved by adding protein to the muscle cells.
15. Testosterone levels influence the degree of size gains.
16. Body type does not influence the degree of size gains.
17. Overload training is necessary in order to achieve size gains.
18. Size gains achieved thru training are permanent.
19. Muscle not used turns to fat.
20. When people stop exercising, they have a tendency to gain weight.
21. A pound of fat is gained by having a positive caloric balance of 3500.
22. Current lifestyles must be balanced with diet to maintain current weight/fat.
23. The average male is stronger than the average female.
24. The average male is bigger than the average female.
25. Skeletal muscle discriminates sexually.
26. Seniors cannot benefit from prudent exercise.
27. Exercise stops the aging process.
28. High intensity exercise is best for seniors.
29. Aging process slows the BMR.
30. The best form of exercise for children is informal spontaneous play.
31. Children cannot be trained above the normal growth curve because of low hormone levels.
32. Exercise in women will always cause an increase in cross sectional size.
33. Exercise in women will always cause an increase in muscle definition.
34. Exercise for women should be discouraged because they will end up looking like a guy.
35. Women have high levels of testosterone.
36. Vitamin supplements are always recommended for college students.
37. Mineral supplements are always recommended for college students.
38. Protein supplements are always recommended for in season athletes.
39. The best supplement is a balanced, mixed diet.
40. Improper use of supplements can be dangerous.

1. _____
2. _____
3. _____
4. _____
5. _____
6. _____
7. _____
8. _____
9. _____
10. _____
11. _____
12. _____
13. _____
14. _____
15. _____
16. _____
17. _____
18. _____
19. _____
20. _____
21. _____
22. _____
23. _____
24. _____
25. _____
26. _____
27. _____
28. _____
29. _____
30. _____
31. _____
32. _____
33. _____
34. _____
35. _____
36. _____
37. _____
38. _____
39. _____
40. _____

CHAPTER NINE
The Value of Warm-Up and Stretching

The preceding chapters have been an introduction to the realm of fitness. They have introduced terms, provided an introduction regarding the function of muscles, explained how the heart operates and provides oxygen to the individual cells and attempted to stimulate an interest in pursuing some increased level of personal fitness. It is anticipated that many questions have been answered and many more have developed. One goal remains, that is to understand the importance of play (fitness activities) for your body. As children, play was essential to all of us. As we have aged, play has taken on new terms, i.e. watching many hours of television, playing video games and eating/hanging out at fast food restaurants. The challenge before you is to bring back play and its positive benefits into your lives. You, the reader must decide the importance of play and becoming more physically active within your life picture. As this choice is made, safe guidelines will help us to establish a well thought out exercise prescription with minimal chance of failure, if your commitment is strong.

The first guideline is to understand the F.I.T. approach, F.I.T. represents frequency, intensity, and time. Frequency indicates how often a workout will be implemented. To maintain average fitness, the recommendation is a minimum of 3 to 5 times a week. With a higher frequency, cross training is recommended to prevent overuse damage to your bodies. Cross training is the incorporation of several activities such as swimming and running to provide the body different challenges every day.

Intensity within aerobic activities is measured through the use of your Target Heart Rate (T.H.R.). The concept has been introduced in an earlier chapter. This is a guideline for safe cardiovascular exercise that is based on age and workload on the heart. Intensity measures within weight training programs are based on sets and reps in defining workload on the muscles involved.

Time is used as a measure of how long the heart must be working at the T.H.R.. With cardiovascular activity, the minimum time of activity should be at least 20 minutes. The 20 minute period starts when the heartrate has reached the Threshold of Training (the lower number of T.H.R.) and remains there. If the activity is sustained less than 20 minutes, the benefit will be increased calorie consumption, although it will have little effect on developing the heart into a stronger, more efficient muscle. For the average American, the length of cardiovascular should not exceed 60 minutes, unless you are training for a specific activity or race.

The second consideration in developing a safe and effective play (fitness) program is to understand the importance of warm-up and stretching. This emphasis on warm-up and stretching is to increase/improve flexibility and prevent possible injury. The new philosophy regarding sequencing of fitness programs is that a warmup should precede all stretching programs. The rationale is that previously warmed up muscles will stretch easier and safer than cold muscles. Therefore warmed-up muscles will have less damage to the muscle fibers.

> **Outside Activity**—Take two rubber bands, take the first rubber band and quickly stretch it as far as possible, you will see damage to the rubber band (be careful not to break the rubber band), take the second rubber band and slowly stretch it out, then relax the stretch, repeat several times. You will notice less damage to the rubber band as the fibers were slowly warmed up. This is a simple demonstration to show the effects on not warming up and stretching your muscle fibers before exercising.

The purpose of all warm-up activity is to slowly increase your heart rate, to increase muscle temperature and to prepare the body for the activity. When discussing warm-up for a team sport, such as basketball, soccer, etc. initiation of shooting, playing catch, moving the ball, and slowly increasing the intensity is appropriate. The days of practice starting with stretching with no previous warm-up activity must be eliminated from sports. With an individual activity, the warm-up should be designed to incorporate the major muscles groups of the body, especially the muscles activity, the warm-up should be designed to incorporate the major muscles groups of the body, especially the muscles that are major contributors to the activity. These activities could include but are not limited to jumping rope, jogging in place, brisk walking, or riding a stationary bicycle. The goals are the same, to gradually elevate the heart rate while raising the temperature of muscle to prepare the muscles for stretching and the physical activity.

The length of the warm-up activity may vary based on weather conditions, psychological attitudes or other physiological concerns. The general rule of thumb is that it should last 5-10 minutes and a light sweat should have been broken. When this has occurred, it is safe to begin the stretching program.

The focus of any stretching program is to prepare the muscles for the activity that will follow and to improve/maintain flexibility. There are three types of stretching programs; ballistic, static, and P.N.F. Of the three types of stretching, the most harmful and dangerous to the body is ballistic. Ballistic stretching is bouncing, where the muscle is stretched quickly and repeatedly. Due to the receptors in the muscle, the muscles work against this quick bounce activity and actually shorten the fibers we are attempting to elongate. This leads to an increase of damage to the musculoskeletal system and is more harmful than good.

Now stand up for a quick demonstration of ballistic stretching. As you are standing with your hands over your head, quickly try and touch your toes. You probably felt a pull in the back of your legs, the hamstring muscle group. That pain or twinge that you felt is the damage being done to the muscle fibers. Ballistic stretching should not be incorporated into any stretching program.

The second type of stretching and most commonly used is static stretching. Static stretching is done at a slow, consistent pace, where the muscles are slowly elongated over each stretch. With static stretching, the muscles are slowly lengthened to the end point. This position is held from 10 to 30 seconds. The process is then repeated several times.

The third manner of stretching is proprioceptive neuromuscular facilitation (PNF) which requires a partner. This stretching technique involves alternating contraction and stretching. PNF has been demonstrated to increase flexibility better than static stretching. The obvious drawback is that a partner had to be involved and that the partner must be well versed in the technique. For most of us we are trying to squeeze some time to workout and we may not have a consistent training partner. That being the case this technique may not be very pratical for us. Improper usage of PNF will lead to muscle damage. PNF technique is more appropriately utilized with athletic teams and therefore will not be addressed any further within this chapter.

Stretching will lead to increased flexibility and lessen any possible muscular damage that may occur from vigorous exercise. It should be incorporated into pre-activity but is also important to incorporate a stretching program into the post-activity session. The rationale for this is that muscles are contracting repeatedly and are becoming tighter by the end of the activity. Therefore, it is highly recommended to perform static stretches at the end of your workout to elongate the muscles. The goal of post-activity stretching is to remove the buildup of lactic acid that occurs with any physical activity. Lactic acid buildup contributes to muscle soreness, so the removal of it through a cool down and stretching is highly beneficial.

The following is a list of guidelines for a safe and beneficial stretching program.

GUIDELINES FOR SAFE AND EFFECTIVE STRETCHING

1. Always precede the stretching program with a limited warmup of 5-10 minutes. Remember that warm muscles elongate better than cold muscles.
2. Always make use of static stretches. They should be slow, easy, with no bounce at all.
3. While stretching, go to the point of mild discomfort and hold. Remain in this position for up to 30 seconds, relax and then repeat several times for each stretch. Each time you stretch you should feel yourself going a little farther.
4. Stretching should be done at least 3-4 times a week. Even if you have to miss an exercise session, try to find the time to stretch and maintain your flexibility.
5. Remember to stretch the major muscle groups, and especially the ones to be used in that fitness activity.
6. Always end your exercise session with a stretching program. This will help reduce muscle soreness and maintain flexibility.

By incorporating a stretching program before and after your fitness activity, there will an increase in flexibility and a lessening of the chance for a serious injury. There are several stretches and activities that are contraindicated (harmful) and should not be considered.

The first one is the straight-leg touch. This is harmful to the low-back, knee and hamstrings. Better choices are utilizing the bent-knee hang. This is done by assuming the same starting position, and then slowly rolling the upper body over. The knees should have a slight bend to them. The upper body is "hanging" and should remain static as you feel the stretch in the hamstring and lower back. An alternative is using a seated stretch, with the knees slightly bent, slowly reaching toward the feet/toes.

A second dangerous stretch-activity is the full squat. A full squat drastically increases the stress placed on the knee and is considered to be very harmful to the knee joint. Squat activities are found in activities such as deep-knee bends, squat thrusts and full squats with weight training. Unfortunately, the full squat is still seen in many weight rooms as the athletes strive to train the full range of motion of the upper leg and gluteal muscles. To decrease the potential danger when performing any squat activity; whether while doing stretching or lifting, the knees should never bend beyond 90 degrees (parallel with the floor).

Another dangerous stretch for the knee is the hurdlers stretch. Here one leg is in front of the body and the other is bent backwards. The stretch occurs as the person attempts to lean back over the back leg. This dramatically increases the stress placed on the knee joint of the back leg. A better and safer stretch is the lateral straddle stretch. In this stretch , the forward leg remains in the same position, but the opposite leg is bent to the side with the foot placed next to the knee of the forward leg (the lower leg will resemble the number 4). The individual then leans forward reaching towards the toes. With this alternative position the stress on the knee has been eliminated.

Other stretches may be dangerous, if any of the following conditions exist or are tried.

1. The joint has more stress placed on it than is normal.
2. There is an over arching of the back and/or neck.
3. The stretch requires a quick bounce.
4. An injury is present and there is limited range of motion due to the injury. When any injury is present it is critical that we listen to our bodies and respond appropriately.

A Basic Stretching Program

Any safe stretching program is designed to include the major muscles of the body: neck, shoulder, arms, back, legs and calves. The goal of the program is to gradually lengthen the muscles and thereby increase range of motion of the joint. Each stretch should be done for up to 30 seconds and should be repeated several times for each muscle.

1. **General Whole Body Stretch**—This is a great beginning stretch that works on the whole body. Lying on the ground, stretch your hands over your head, stretch your legs down in the opposite direction of the arms. Make yourself longer. While doing this stretch, it is important to breathe very slowly and deeply.
2. **Neck Stretch**—Grasp the back of your head and/ or the opposite side of the head and use your hand to pull the head gently to the side and to the front. Switch hands to stretch the opposite direction.
3. **Chest and Arms**—Stand sideways to a wall/doorway at arms length. Reach out and slightly behind you and place the palm on the wall. While holding the palm on the wall, turn your body away from the wall as far as your body allows. Remember to keep the arm at 90 degrees to the body and keep your hips touching the wall as you rotate. Repeat several times and switch arms.
4. **Shoulders and Upper Back**—While sitting or standing, place the right palm behind your neck onto the right shoulder. With the left hand, grasp the right elbow and pull it slowly behind you. Another variation is to bring your left hand up behind the back and grasp your right hand. After grasping your right hand slowly pull down. Hold and relax, repeat several times and then switch sides. This position is also used to test shoulder flexibility.
5. **Lower Back Stretches**—Lie flat on your back and bring one knee up to your chest. Hold onto the upper leg, while keeping the other leg on the floor with the knee slightly bent. Place gentle pressure on the leg towards the chest and curl your head up toward the knee. Hold, relax and repeat several times with each leg.
6. **Another Low Back Stretch**—While lying flat on your back, bring both of your knees up to your chest, grasp them with your hands and curl your head up towards the chest. Again, relax, and repeat several times.
7. **Hamstring Stretch** (previously described as the lateral stretch)—While sitting on the floor, with one leg extended, the opposite knee is bent with the foot touching the extended leg's knee. Then while keeping your back straight, bend at the hips (not shoulders) and reach for your toes. Remember to keep the extended leg slightly bent. Repeat several times and switch to the other leg.
8. **Adductor Stretch**—Often referred as the butterfly stretch. While in a sitting position on the floor, bend both knees and place the soles of the feet together at the groin elbow. While holding on to the ankles, bend at the hips and place the elbows on the knees. You will use your body weight to place pressure and stretch the inner thighs. Hold, relax and repeat several times.

9. **Calf Muscle Stretch**—While standing facing a wall, from approximately arms length, lean towards the wall. You must keep your heels on the ground, legs straight and support your weight with the hands.
10. **Press Up**—An additional activity that needs to be introduced. The press up should be used after every abdominal exercise to help realign the back. When crunches are incorporated into our fitness regime they tend to leave the back (spinal column) in a tight position. By using press ups, we can help with the repositioning and adjustment of the spinal column. After all abdominal work, remember to do 10 press ups.

By incorporating some or all of these actions into both a pre and post-activity stretching program, the individual will be on the road to increased flexibility. Remember to follow the guidelines presented within this chapter and only compare your flexibility to yourself. As with all fitness activities, each person has different abilities and he/she should not compete with anyone else. With the majority of fitness pursuits, we are only competing against ourself and increasing our fitness level.

TREATMENT FOR BASIC FITNESS RELATED INJURIES
Within the presentation of flexibility and the discussion of the value of stretching, it was mentioned that increased flexibility will help reduce the severity of injury. At this point, it is appropriate to introduce the fact that with fitness pursuits, there exists a risk of injury, and we should have a basic knowledge of fitness injuries. The cause of these injuries run the gamut from overuse, overtraining, poor technique to just the unfortunate ankle sprains due to a pothole on your favorite training route. With any injury, we must know the appropriate immediate first aid and be concerned with the deconditioning that will occur as a result. Many injuries will not preclude us from all fitness activities, but we may have to make appropriate changes in our fitness program.

The easiest manner to deal with injury is prevention. Many fitness related injuries could be easily prevented by following some basic guidelines, such as using proper equipment and listening to your body. Injuries used to be seen as major setbacks, where all activity must cease. As sports medicine specialists have become more available to the general public, many more injuries are being treated with a more progressive approach. This allows the injured person to continue with other reasonable and safe pursuits while allowing for rest and healing to occur at the injury site. This philosophy slows the deconditioning process down and allows the injured person to better maintain his/her mental and physical edge through modified activity.

The appropriate treatment for all acute (sudden onset) injuries is known as R.I.C.E. (Rest, Ice, Compression, Elevation). This should be applied as soon as possible after the initial determination of severity. Never under any circumstance should heat be used as the treatment for any acute injury. The application of cold therapy is suggested for the first 72 hours, and the ice should be applied for periods of 20 minutes, then removed for 30 minutes before it is reapplied.

How does RICE work and what are the physiological changes that occur when applied to an acute injury? Rest literally means to stop what you are doing. Continued usage could cause further damage to the involved area. Depending on the severity of the injury, after the 20 minutes of ice the individual may be able to begin participating again.

Ice causes constriction of the vascular system (arteries and veins that circulate blood), thereby lessening the bloodflow out of the vascular system and into the injury site. This assists in controlling edema and swelling to the area. The other effect of ice is the numbing effect that reduces the pain level of the injured person.

Compression works in conjunction with the ice in decreasing the blood flow and lessening the leakage of blood to the injured area. Often the seriousness of an injury is not specifically related to the damage to the ligaments, muscle or tendons, but more to the level of swelling occurring at the injury site. This swelling may cause restriction and impede the function of the joint/muscles.

Elevation of the injured body part is the last component in decreasing swelling and pain at the injury. Elevation of the injury should always be above the heart. Elevation of the body part allows gravity to slow the flow of blood to the injury, thereby lessening the amount of blood flowing past and leaking out.

After the initial treatment of RICE has been applied, options/questions still may remain. These questions relate to the seriousness of the injury. Does it require immediate medical attention? Is weight bearing tolerated? How much pain exists? Can we continue to exercise? Remember to use common sense. If pain exists then you are probably not ready to continue your program. And if there are any doubts, see your doctor.

CLASSIFICATIONS OF INJURIES
The majority of fitness related injuries involve the musculoskeletal system. These include contusions of soft tissue, strains to the musculotendinous unit (often referred to as a pulled muscle), ligamentous sprains, fractures and overuse injuries.

Contusions are commonly caused from a direct blow by another object or person that damages the soft tissue surrounding the injury site. The damage is localized bleeding which may "pool" below the injury site due to the effects of gravity. Contusions are not often serious, but may limit activity for several days.

Muscle strains are known as a pulled muscle. The damage occurs and inflammation begins when the skeletal muscle or tendon fibers start to separate. This injury is often caused by sudden explosive muscular contractions, lack of flexibility or a muscle imbalance. Muscle strains are very common in the larger muscle groups of the body—quadriceps, hamstrings, groin, pectorals and biceps.

Sprains are damage to ligaments, which are the connective tissues between articulating bones. The mechanisms of injury for sprains are often a twisting action, turning the joint over, or any excessive force applied to the joint.

Fractures occur less often in fitness activities than in sport and are often secondary to "bad luck" or careless behavior. Whenever a snap, crack or pop is heard, be aware that the force of the injury has the potential for a fracture. The noise you hear may be bone rubbing on bone, the ligament tearing, or bone breaking. The injured person in this case should take the precaution of contacting their Doctor and having X-rays for a definitive medical diagnosis.

The last classification of injuries and probably the most common occurrence in fitness pursuits are overuse injuries. Overuse injuries have the suffix "itis" at the end, which indicates inflammation of the body part. Overuse injuries usually develop gradually through the repetitive nature of endurance activities. These injuries are hard to evaluate because the onset of pain is gradual and often described as a dull, throbbing ache. If they are ignored, overuse injuries usually develop into more serious and long lasting problems. When an individual has a gradual onset of pain from an unknown source, he/she should discontinue the fitness activity, use RICE and have it evaluated by a qualified sports medicine practitioner.

FINAL THOUGHTS

The goals of this chapter were to provide the framework for beginning a safe, successful fitness program. Within this framework, the discussion was centered on the importance of beginning all fitness activities with a warm-up session. The importance of a warm-up is to provide the body with an opportunity to prepare the systems of the body for exercise. The next topic discussed was a safe stretching program that should be incorporated before and at the end of all exercise programs. The value of stretching is to increase the body's flexibility and reduce the seriousness of injury.

The chapter ends with an introduction regarding basic injury care and terminology for the lay person. The best recommendation that can be made to all those who increase their play programs is to listen to your body. If your body is sore or in pain, then modifications must be made to your program to allow the body a time period to heal itself. The usage of RICE will most likely shorten the recovery time of most minor injuries. The other important aspect regarding injury is that your fitness plan does not have to come to a complete standstill. The concept of cross-training or making modifications to your current program is highly recommended. Get in the pool, on the bike, whatever is reasonable and doesn't increase the pain at the injury site.

WORKSHEET 9-A

Chapter Nine—The Value of Warm-up, Stretching and Basic Injury Care

Matching: Put the letter of the definition next to the term/phrase.

Terms/Phrases

1. F.I.T. Principle
2. F. of the F.I.T.
3. I. of the F.I.T.
4. T. of the F.I.T.
5. Warm Up
6. Ballistic Stretch
7. Static Stretch
8. PNF Stretch
9. 30 Seconds
10. Straight Leg touch
11. Full Squat
12. Hurdlers Stretch
13. R.i.C.E. Principle
14. R. of R.I.C.E.
15. I. of R.I.C.E.
16. C. of R.I.C.E.
17. E. of R.I.C.E.
18. Contusions
19. Strains
20. Sprains
21. Fractures
22. "ITIS"
23. Press up
24. Overuse injury
25. 72 hours

1. _____
2. _____
3. _____
4. _____
5. _____
6. _____
7. _____
8. _____
9. _____
10. _____
11. _____
12. _____
13. _____
14. _____
15. _____
16. _____
17. _____
18. _____
19. _____
20. _____
21. _____
22. _____
23. _____
24. _____
25. _____

Definitions

A. Repetitive trauma to a body part.
B. Inflammation of a body part as a result of trauma.
C. Over stretching of a ligament.
D. Soft tissue damage from a direct impact.
E. Compression of the injury site to reduce swelling.
F. Resting phase of injury treatment.
G. Dangerous stretch of the knee by leaning back.
H. Dangerous stretch to low back.
I. Proprioneuromuscular Facilitation stretching.
J. Bobbing or bouncing stretch.
K. The recommended length of time of an exercise bout.

L.   The recommended frequency of exercise bouts.

M.   Length of time ice should be used after an injury.

N.   Exercise that helps to realign the vertebral column.

O.   Actual breaking of a bone.

P.   Muscular injury from overintensity.

Q.   Elevating an injured body part to assist drainage & reduce swelling.

R.   Ice application to reduce the general adverse effects of the trauma.

S.   Standard injury treatment protocol.

T.   Dangerous exercise that over stretches the knee joint.

U.   Length of time a static stretch should be held.

V.   Stretching a body part slowly & then holding the stretch position.

W.   General exercise protocol that prepares the body for high intensity action.

X.   Intensity of the workout bout measured by heart rate.

Y.   Standard exercise protocol for frequency, intensity & time.

CHAPTER TEN
Aerobic and Anaerobic Exercise

The word aerobic means with air or oxygen. The human body is an aerobic body since it must have a continuous supply of oxygen. Any cells in the body that are deprived of oxygen die. Exercise has been divided into two categories, aerobic and anaerobic, based upon the amount of oxygen available for energy production.

METABOLISM

The first law of thermodynamics is that energy is neither created or destroyed but is transferred from one form to another. Metabolism is the conversion of chemical energy to mechanical energy.

The human body requires mechanical energy to carry out it's many processes. Mechanical energy can be defined as the ability to do work. Some examples of how the body uses mechanical energy are digestion, nerve transmission, circulation and building tissues. The principle role of mechanical energy, from the exercise perspective, is muscle contraction.

Chemical energy in food nutrients is changed to mechanical energy by the action of the musculoskeletal system. The conversion of this energy from glucose, fat and protein molecules usually occurs in the presence of oxygen. For this reason the body must continually supply fuel (food nutrients) and oxygen to the tissues.

METABOLIC NEEDS

Metabolism at rest is called the basal metabolic rate (BMR). When the body changes from a resting state to a working state additional mechanical energy is required. This requires additional fuel (food nutrients, carbohydrates, fat and protein) and oxygen. The heart rate will increase to move these stored fuel sources to the functioning muscle cells. The breathing rate will increase also, as additional oxygen is needed for the conversion of chemical energy to mechanical energy. Metabolic rate is determined by the amount of work that the body has to do (metabolic needs). Metabolism is measured by oxygen consumption.

> What determines your metabolic rate?
> _____

There are times when the body is forced to work at an accelerated rate. Often the cardiorespiratory system is unable to take in and circulate enough oxygen to provide for the conversion of chemical energy to mechanical energy. The body has the capacity to generate mechanical energy with insufficient amounts of oxygen. This is a short term process of under two minutes. It is called anaerobic metabolism.

AEROBIC EXERCISE

Some aerobic activities are walking, jogging, swimming, cycling, and cross country skiing. Aerobic exercise is characterized as large muscle, rhythmic, prolonged activity.

The most common muscle groups used in aerobic exercise are the leg muscles. Arm muscles are also used in some cases and at other times a combination of arms and legs are used. Aerobic exercise is performed at a steady pace (rhythmic) and at less than maximal effort. At maximal effort the cardiorespiratory system cannot provide the oxygen needed for aerobic metabolism to occur.

To provide conditioning for the cardiovascular system, aerobic exercise must be continued for a prolonged period of time. A minimal duration is twelve minutes with twenty minute sessions providing far better results.

Any activity can be classified as aerobic if the energy requirement remains below the level at which the body can continue to convert chemical energy to mechanical energy in the presence of oxygen. Some additional examples of good aerobic activities are aerobic dance, step aerobics, stair climbing, rowing and dancing.

ANAEROBIC EXERCISE

When the intensity of exercise is at a very high rate, the body may not be able to provide an adequate oxygen supply for the conversion of chemical energy. The body has the capacity to generate energy without an adequate oxygen supply. This process is called anaerobic metabolism. When metabolism occurs without adequate oxygen, large amounts of lactic acid are created. If this high intensity exercise is prolonged, the oxygen debt increases as does the build up lactic acid. This will ultimately require a cessation or slow down of the activity. Typical anaerobic exercise involves all out effort in short bursts. Some examples of anaerobic exercise include sprinting, weight lifting, and racquetball.

All individuals have an anaerobic capacity. Duration is usually something less than two minutes. The length is determined by individual physiological characteristics and anaerobic training.

A result of inadequate warm-up is that when you begin to exercise you will experience anaerobic metabolism. The body is being required to go directly from a resting state to a working state. This requires the production of additional energy. The body provides this anaerobically. Gradually as you continue the work the pulmonary and cardiovascular systems speed up their circulation of oxygen to the tissues, and energy production returns to an aerobic state. This condition is often referred to as "second wind". It is the point at which energy production becomes aerobic.

A common method for determining the intensity of the workout is to count the exercise heart rate. Since the initial work is often anaerobic, the heart rate will be irregular until you reach the aerobic state. Therefore, for a valid determination of intensity, one should wait until at least four minutes into the workout before checking their heart rate.

AEROBIC PROGRAM DESIGN

Before entering an aerobic fitness program one should determine their current health status. If one is under 35 years of age, in good health and with a good family history for cardiovascular disease, they should be able to enter into an aerobic fitness program without a medical exam. Persons who do not meet these criteria should get permission from their physician before entering the program.

It is also important to determine the currant fitness status before starting a fitness program. Fitness testing will provide the individual with an evaluation of their personal capability. There are fitness tests for all health and skill related components of fitness. It is usually beneficial to have a comprehensive fitness assessment. This chapter will address an evaluation of cardiovascular endurance.

There are several methods of measuring cardiovascular fitness. When determining the test to be used, one should consider the mode of aerobic training that they will participate in. The law of specificity is that the mode of testing and training should be the same. In one study, two groups entered an aerobic fitness program. Both groups were tested on cycle ergometers and treadmills. One group cycled for training while the other group jogged. When retested the jogging group showed significant improvement in both the cycle ergometer and treadmill tests. The cycling group only showed significant improvement in the cycle ergometer test. Improvements tend to be specific to the training mode. This is due to the training of muscular strength, cardiovascular endurance and the development of neural pathways. Based on this law of specificity, one should decide how they want to train before they select a testing mode.

A second consideration to be made is the accuracy that is required. The most accurate methods involve the use of electrocardiographic monitoring and the collection and analysis of exhaled air. These tests can be done while running on a treadmill or riding a cycle ergometer. Very sophisticated and expensive equipment is required. Trained professionals are needed to administer and monitor the testing apparatus. Because of these facts, and that the test must be administered to one individual at a time, the cost of testing is high.

A final consideration is the methods of testing that are available. If a testing lab is unavailable, a field test can be used to provide the necessary information. Some examples of field tests of cardiovascular fitness are:

12 Minute Running Test
1 1/2 Mile Running Test
Bench Stepping Tests

Each of these tests will determine the body's ability to take in, circulate and use oxygen to release energy. The running tests measure the individual's ability to run as far or as fast as they can for an extended period of time. The bench stepping tests are usually shorter in duration and measure the individual's recovery heart rate from the work session.

Rate your level of cardiovascular fitness. (Superior, Excellent, Good, Fair, Poor, Very Poor)

INDIVIDUALIZED PROGRAMS

Nearly every individual has a different capacity for performing aerobic fitness exercise. A program must be designed to meet the specific needs of each person. If a person trains at a level that is too difficult, the risk of injury increases. A result of difficult exercise is that one may encounter a good deal of pain and discomfort during and after exercise. Most people do not enjoy or choose to participate in unpleasant activities. Therefore the result is high program dropout rates.

Conversely, if the exercise program is not difficult enough for the person they will not see a change in their cardiovascular endurance. Few people will choose to participate in an exercise program that provides little or no benefit.

It is also important to select activities that the individual enjoys. It is difficult to participate in an activity that one does not enjoy. A final consideration is the availability of the activity. Studies have shown that the most common reason for quitting an exercise program is that it is not convenient from either a time or travel standpoint.

OVERLOAD PRINCIPLE

To provide physical training for the human body an exercise program must follow the "overload principle". This applies, not only to weight training programs but, to all types of physical training. The principle requires that the cardiovascular system must be stressed beyond the point that it habitually encounters. As the body gradually gains in cardiovascular conditioning, the initial program will no longer be adequate to improve aerobic fitness. It will only maintain the present level. Only a program of progressive resistance that overloads the cardiovascular system will provide for improvements in cardiovascular endurance.

The individualized aerobic fitness program will use the entry test results to identify the initial workload for the program. Progressive increases must be made as one continues the program. When the load is increased the body responds with an increased capacity to do physical work. When one reaches the level of fitness that they desire, they can cease to increase the workload. If they continue to work at a constant workload they will maintain their current level of fitness.

WORKOUT COMPONENTS

Any workout should be composed of three parts: warm up, workout activity and cool down. The warm-up session prepares the body for the vigorous physical work to be encountered. Stretching exercises should be the second part of the warm-up and help to prepare the body for the activity. Chapter 9 provides details on the warm-up and cool down procedure. In aerobic fitness programs, the warm-up should include a short period of the selected activity at a slower than normal pace. This helps to ease the cardiovascular system into the work. After the exercise activity is completed the cool down exercises will gradually help to return the body to it's resting state. Stretching exercises should be the final stage of a workout.

EXERCISE PROGRAMS

An aerobic fitness program should be designed around four principles. These are intensity, duration, frequency and mode. These four principles will be explained in Chapter 11.

Exercise Equipment

Selection of proper equipment is important in aerobic training programs. The old saying "no pain no gain" has little merit. There is no question that to have value exercise must involve hard work. This does not mean that you need to push yourself to the limit every time you work out. Proper dress for the chosen activity can have a substantial impact on the avoidance of discomfort.

Selecting good aerobic equipment can serve two important roles. New exercise clothing or shoes can motivate the participant to sustain their interest. It also reduces the risk of injury.

Walking/Jogging

Both walking and jogging programs involve activity where the body weight must be supported by the feet and legs. This suggests that the most important equipment for these two activities is good footwear.

Walking programs are far less demanding on the feet and legs than are jogging programs. One must have a pair of shoes that are comfortable. A major injury that occurs from ill fitting footwear is blisters. It is for this reason that a proper shoe fit is important. If you find that you must purchase shoes there are shoes that are specifically designed for exercise walking programs.

Jogging programs require good running shoes. The shoe that is required is called a training flat. This shoe is constructed specifically for the constant shock experienced from jogging. Racing flats, basketball or aerobic shoes are not designed for this purpose. A very common cause of many foot and leg injuries is poor footwear. Jogging shoes should have good flexibility in the forefoot. This is where your foot has to bend when you push off. Many less expensive shoes have very poor flexibility. The heal of the shoe should be higher than the forefoot. Most shoes have two or three layers of composition material that becomes thicker toward the heel of the shoe.

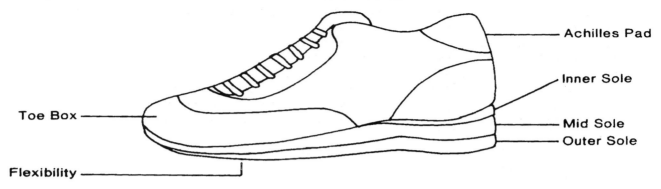

Figure 10-1

Dress for outdoor exercise must take into account the weather conditions and the amount of heat the body will generate during the exercise activity. The higher the intensity level the more heat that will be generated by the body. In cool weather, the excess body heat can be used to keep the body warm. Where as in warm weather, this excess heat causes the body to become overheated.

In warm weather the rule is to expose the skin to the air. The bodies cooling system works by moving heat to the surface of the body; where perspiration helps to dissapate the heat into the atmosphere. White shorts and t-shirts or tank tops are ideal for warm weather exercise. Wool socks are good since they will wick moisture away from the feet. In bright sun a white hat will reflect sun light.

When the weather is cooler in spring or fall, a long sleeved shirt and sweat pants help to maintain some body heat. In these seasons rain is common. There are water proof suits that are designed to keep you dry. The fact is that they keep the rain out but also keep heat in and cause you to perspire. The perspiration is trapped inside the rain suit, and you get wet from perspiration instead of the rain. A wind breaker will not keep the rain out but it does help to keep heat in. Since you will get wet with either, the wind breaker that is far less expensive is the best choice. Getting wet is not a problem unless you get cold. This can be prevented by moving inside immediately after your workout.

Indoor Exercise Programs

Aerobic Dance and step aerobics will require good exercise shoes. Other activities such as rowing, stairclimbing and cycling do not put undo stress on the feet and legs and thus the need for good quality footwear is reduced.

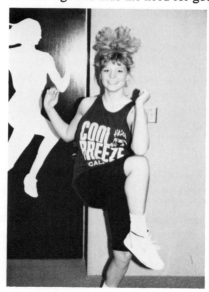

Figure 10-2

74

All of these activities require comfortable dress. Many who participate in aerobic exercise have colorful tights but equal benefit can be achieved with any other comfortable clothing.

SUMMARY

Aerobic activities are those activities that are done at less than maximal capacity, at a steady pace and for a prolonged period of time. Energy is provided in the presence of oxygen.

Anaerobic activities are done at a high intensity level, usually at maximum capacity for short periods of time. Energy is provided with a less than adequate oxygen supply.

In this chapter you have learned the importance of entry level testing and how it affects the design of individualized exercise programs. The "overload principle" and progressive resistance have been defined as the methods used for the development of his/her levels of fitness. Specificity of exercise is important to ensure that your exercise mode will produce the desired results. The exercise session has been discussed as to warm-up, activity and cool down.

Footwear is the most important equipment needed for most exercise programs. Outdoor exercise must take weather conditions into consideration.

WORKSHEET 10-A

Chapter Ten—Aerobic and Anaerobic Exercise

True/False

1. Aerobic means with oxygen.   1. _____
2. Anaerobic means without oxygen.   2. _____
3. Cells deprived of oxygen live about two weeks.   3. _____
4. Metabolism is the conversion of chemical to mechanical energy.   4. _____
5. An example of chemical energy is food nutrients.   5. _____
6. An example of mechanical energy is walking.   6. _____
7. Basal Metabolic Rate (BMR) is the resting energy level.   7. _____
8. Any increase in activity causes an elevation of the BMR.   8. _____
9. The higher the activity level, the higher the BMR goes.   9. _____
10. The higher the BMR goes, the more calories are burned.   10. _____
11. The more at rest the body is, the fewer calories it burns.   11. _____
12. Sprinting and power lifting are examples of aerobic exercise. 12. _____
13. Jogging and swimming are examples of anaerobic exercise.   13. _____
14. Aerobic exercise primarily trains the skeletal muscles.   14. _____
15. Anaerobic exercise primarily trains the cardiovascular system. 15. _____
16. The 12 minute test measure cardiofitness.   16. _____
17. The mile and a half run measures cardiofitness.   17. _____
18. Bench stepping measures leg power.   18. _____
19. Fitness programs should be personalized.   19. _____
20. Enjoyment of the exercise enhances compliance to the program. 20. _____
21. The Overload Principle means a gradual increase of the workload. 21. _____
22. Improvements in fitness are directly correlated to the work done. 22. _____
23. Quality, well fitted athletic shoes are essential.   23. _____
24. It is not necessary to warm up prior to an aerobic workout.   24. _____
25. It is not necessary to cool down after an aerobic workout.   25. _____

WORKSHEET 10B
MEN'S AEROBICS FITNESS CLASSIFICATION (PREDICTED)   Score _____

CATEGORY	MEASURE	13-19	20-29	30-39	Age (years) 40-49	50-59	60+
I. Very poor	O_2 uptake (ml/kg/min.)	<35.0	<33.0	<31.5	<30.2	<26.1	<20.5
	*T.M. time (min.:sec.)	<14:30	<12:50	<12:00	<11:00	<9:00	<5:30
	12-min. dist. (mile)	<1.30	<1.22	<1:18	<1.14	<1.03	<.87
	1.5-mile time (min.:sec.)	>15:31	>16:01	>16:31	>17.31	>19:01	>20:01
II. Poor	O_2 uptake (ml/kg/min.)	35.0-38.3	33.0-36.4	31.5-35.4	30.2-33.5	26.1-30.9	20.5-26.0
	*T.M. time (min.:sec.)	14:30-16:44	12:50-15:29	12:00-14:59	11:00-13:29	9:00-11:29	5:30-8:49
	12-min. dist. (mile)	1.30-1.37	1.22-1.31	1.18-1.30	1.14-1.24	1.03-1.16	.87-1.02
	1.5-mile time (min.:sec.)	12:11-15:30	14:01-16:00	14:44-16:30	15:36-17:30	17:01-19:00	19:01-20:00
III. Fair	O_2 uptake (ml/kg/min.)	38.4-45.1	36.5-42.4	35.5-40.9	33.6-38.9	31.0-35.7	26.1-32.2
	*T.M. time (min.:sec.)	16:45-21:07	15:30-18:59	15:00-17:59	13:30-16:59	11:30-14:59	8:50-12:29
	12-min. dist. (mile)	1.38-1.56	1.32-1.49	1.31-1.45	1.25-1.39	1.17-1.30	1.03-1.20
	1.5-mile time (min.:sec.)	10:49-12:10	12:01-14:00	12:31-14.45	13:01-15:35	14:31-17:00	16:16-19:00
IV. Good	O_2 uptake (ml/kg/min.)	45.2-50.9	42.5-46.4	41.0-44.9	39.0-43.7	35.8-40.9	32.2-36.4
	*T.M. time (min.:sec.)	21:08-24:44	19:00-21:59	18:00-20:59	17:00-19:59	15:00-17:59	12:30-15:44
	12-min. dist. (mile)	1.57-1.72	1.5-1.64	1.46-1.56	1.40-1.53	1.31-1.44	1.21-1.32
	1.5-mile time (min.:sec.)	9:41-10:48	10:46-12:00	11:01-12:30	11:31-13:00	12:31-14:30	14:00-16:15
V. Excellent	O_2 uptake (ml/kg/min.)	51.0-55.9	46.5-52.4	45.0-49.4	43.8-48.0	41.0-45.3	36.5-44.2
	*T.M. time (min.:sec.)	24:45-27:47	22:00-24:59	21:00-23:59	20:00-22:59	18:00-21:14	15:45-20:37
	12-min. dist. (mile)	1.73-1.86	1.65-1.76	1.57-1.69	1.54-1.65	1.45-1.58	1.33-1.55
	1.5-mile time (min.:sec.)	8:37-9:40	9:45-10:45	10:00-11:00	10:30-11:30	11:00-12:30	11:15-13:59
VI. Superior	O_2 uptake (ml/kg/min.)	>56.0	>52.5	>49.5	>48.1	>45.4	>44.3
	*T.M. time (min.:sec.)	>27:48	>25:00	>24:00	>23:00	>21.:15	>20:38
	12-min. dist. (mile)	>1.87	>1.77	>1.70	>1.56	>1.59	>1.56
	1.5-mile time (min.:sec.)	<8:37	<9:45	<10:00	<10:30	<11:00	<11:15

WOMEN'S AEROBICS FITNESS CLASSIFICATION (PREDICTED)   Score _____

CATEGORY	MEASURE	13-19	20-29	30-39	Age (years) 40-49	50-59	60+
I. Very poor	O_2 uptake (ml/kg/min.)	<25.0	<23.6	<22.8	<21.0	<20.2	<17.5
	*T.M. time (min.:sec.)	<8:30	<7:46	<7:15	<6:00	<5:38	<4:00
	12-min. dist. (mile)	<1.0	<.96	<.96	<.94	<.88	<.84	<.78
	1.5-mile time (min.:sec.)	>18:31	>19.01	>19:31	>20:01	>20:31	>21.01
II. Poor	O_2 uptake (ml/kg/min.)	25.0-30.9	23.6-28.9	22.8-26.9	21.0-24.4	20.2-22.7	17.5-20.1
	*T.M. time (min.:sec.)	8:30-11:29	7:46-10:09	7:15-9:29	6:00-7:59	5:38-6:59	4:00-5:32
	12-min. dist. (mile)	1.00-1.18	.96-1.11	.95-1.05	.88-.98	.84-.93	.78-.86
	1.5-mile time (min.:sec.)	18:30-16:55	19:00-18:31	19:30-19:01	20:00-19:31	20.30-20.01	21:00-20:31
III. Fair	O_2 uptake (ml/kg/min.)	31.0-34.9	29.0-32.9	27.0-31.4	24.5-28.9	22.8-26.9	20.2-24.4
	*T.M. time (min.:sec.)	11:30-13:59	10:10-12:59	9:30-11:59	8:00-10:59	7:00-9:29	5:33-7:59
	12-min. dist. (mile)	1.19-1.29	1.12-1.22	1.06-1.18	.99-1.11	.94-1.05	.87-.98
	1.5-mile time (min.:sec.)	16:54-14:31	18:30-15:55	19:00-16:31	19:30-17:31	20:00-19:01	20:30-19:31
IV. Good	O_2 uptake (ml/kg/min.)	35.0-38.9	33.0-36.9	31.5-35.6	29.0-32.8	27.0-31.4	24.5-30.2
	*T.M. time (min.:sec.)	14:00-17:29	13:00-15:59	12:00-14:59	11:00-12:59	9:30-11:59	8:00-10:59
	12-min. dist. (mile)	1.30-1.43	1.23-1.34	1.19-1.29	1.12-1.24	1.06-1.18	.99-1.09
	1.5-mile time (min.:sec.)	14:30-12:30	15:54-13.31	16:30-14:31	17:30-15:56	19:00-16:31	19:30-17:31
V. Excellent	O_2 uptake (ml/kg/min.)	39.0-41.9	37.0-40.9	35.7-40.0	32.9-36.9	31.5-35.7	30.3-31.4
	*T.M. time (min.:sec.)	17:30-18:59	16:00-17:59	15:00-16:59	13:00-15:59	12:00-14:59	11:00-11:59
	12-min. dist. (mile)	1.44-1.51	1.35-1.45	1.30-1.39	1.25-1.34	1.19-1.30	1.10-1.18
	1.5-mile time (min.:sec.)	12:29-11:50	13:30-12:30	14:30-13:00	15:55-13:45	16:30-14:30	17:30-16:30
VI. Superior	O_2 uptake (ml/kg/min.)	>42.0	>41.0	>40.1	>37.0	>35.8	>31.5
	*T.M. time (min.:sec.)	>19:00	>18:00	>17:00	>16:00	>15:00	>12:00
	12-min. dist. (mile)	>1.52	>1.46	>1.40	>1.35	>1.31	>1.19
	1.5-mile time (min.:sec.)	<11:50	<12:30	<13:00	<13:45	<14:30	<16:30

*Treadmill time using Balke-Ware technique.

From *The Aerobics Way* by Kenneth H. Cooper. Copyright © 1977 by Kenneth H. Cooper. Used by permission of Bantam Books, a division of Bantam Doubleday Dell Publishing Group, Inc.

CHAPTER ELEVEN
Aerobic Training Principles

Many people who start an exercise program do it to improve their health. After several months in an exercise program, most will tell you that they exercise because it makes them feel good. This is a large part of the motivating force that keeps them going. It is difficult to measure feeling good, but easy to measure the physiological changes that occur due to regular exercise. Physical changes such as improved muscular strength, muscular endurance, cardiovascular endurance, flexibility and body composition can be readily measured.

Success in a fitness program will depend upon two major conditions. The first is that you start slowly and progress at a gradual pace. The second condition is that you must follow closely the prescribed program established for your chosen activity.

Far too many people start an exercise program with the idea that they will work hard and regain their lost level of fitness in a week or two. When this doesn't happen they become discouraged and quit. Remember, it took many weeks to become deconditioned, and you cannot regain a high level of physical fitness in a few days. Poor technique often leads to injuries. Pain and discomfort are good motivators to cause you to quit your exercise program.

This chapter will detail the procedure for designing various aerobic fitness programs. It will identify proper technique for implementation of several aerobic activities. It also will examine the physiological changes that result from aerobic training.

The design of a successful aerobic fitness program will require that four variables be addressed. These are intensity, duration, frequency and mode.

MODE

The first decision will be what mode of exercise should be used. The mode of exercise simply means what exercise activities are you going to do. As has been mentioned before, the most important factors are activities that will not only improve your fitness, but will be enjoyable and are convenient for you.

Jogging and walking are popular choices because they require little equipment and no special facilities. Cycling requires either a bicycle or an ergometer and little else. Swimming requires a pool that may not be conveniently located. Cross country skiing requires snow or Nordic Ski equipment. Aerobic exercise sessions require audio or video tapes or an instructor and groups of people. Classes with instructors are also usually scheduled at specific hours at specific location which may or may not fit into your schedule.

There are other modes of aerobic training that can be used such as rowers and stairclimbers or circuit weight training. Each requires special equipment.

It is important to note that the mode will not determine the fitness outcome. One can gain very good aerobic fitness using any of these modes of exercise. The key issue is regular participation at appropriate intensity and duration levels.

INTENSITY

Once you have selected an activity, you must determine how hard you have to perform this activity. This is called the intensity of the program. It addresses how fast you should run, walk, cycle or swim. The controlling factor is that cardiovascular endurance programs use the aerobic training procedure. This requires large muscle, rhythmic and prolonged activity. The above activities use large muscle groups. Each of these activities should be done at a specific pace that is continued for a prolonged period of time. One should set an intensity pace that they can continued for the duration of the program. If this occurs, the exercise heart rate will remain the same throughout the session. This meets the rhythmic requirement. The prolonged activity factor will be addressed later.

The intensity of the program must be maintained within the aerobic capacity of the individual. One must attain an intensity level that will provide cardiovascular conditioning. Due to it's relationship to aerobic capacity, the easiest method to establish an intensity level is by monitoring the heart rate. The rule is that the lower limits of exercise should be established at sixty percent of maximum capacity. Upper limits should not exceed ninety percent of maximum capacity.

One can only know their true maximum capacity (heart rate) if they have had a monitored cardiovascular test to exhaustion. Without this test an estimate of maximum heart rate must be used. The process for estimating maximum heart rate is as follows.

Formula	220 - Age = Estimated Maximum Heart Rate
Example	220 - 20 years = 200 Maximum Heart Rate

Whether using the actual or estimated maximum heart rate, the process for establishing the intensity range of the exercise program is as follows.

Formula
        Lower Limit = Maximum Heart Rate X Minimum Percent
        Upper Limit = Maximum Heart Rate X Maximum Percent
Example
        Lower Limit = 200 X 60 % = 120 Beats Per Minute (B/M)
        Upper Limit = 200 X 90 % = 180 Beats Per Minute (B/M)

This tells us that the intensity level of the aerobic fitness program for a 20 year old should raise the heart rate to a minimum level of 120 B/M but not exceed 180 B/M. If the heart rate is lower than 120 B/M, there will be little if any conditioning of the cardiovascular system. If the heart rate exceeds 180 B/M, the individual will cross over into anaerobic training. This will result in a reduction in the duration of the program.

This formula will apply regardless of the level of conditioning at entry into the program. This is true since the more deconditioned person will have a higher heart rate at lower speeds than will trained persons. As cardiovascular endurance develops, the heart rate will rise more slowly and higher intensity work will be required to maintain the heart rate within the prescribed limits. This is an example of the implementation of the "overload principle."

The best method for monitoring the exercise heart rate is to stop and check your pulse. This can be done by monitoring the radial or carotid pulse. The best time is four to five minutes into the exercise session. Try to find the pulse quickly and count it for ten seconds. Multiply this number by six to calculate your heart rate for one minute. This is made easier by calculating your ten second heart rate range before you begin exercising. This is done as follows.

Formula
        Lower Level Heart Rate/6 = Minimum 10 Second Rate
        Upper Level Heart Rate/6 = Maximum 10 Second Rate

Example
        120/6 = 20
        180/6 = 30

By following this procedure, a 20 year old will know that their ten second exercise pulse should be between 20 and 30 B/M.

Another method of measuring the intensity of an aerobic exercise program is called perceived exertion. This process requires the individual to estimate how hard they are working by how they feel. This method works very well for experienced exercisers. As you progress in the exercise program you learn how you feel when your heart rate is at different levels during their workout. The process is much less effective with new exercisers, since it is difficult for them to comprehend what they should feel like when they are exercising.

A third method of determining intensity when running is called the "talk method." If your intensity level is appropriate, you should be able to carry on a conversation with a running partner. You will normally have to use shorter phrases but it should not be labored.

It is more difficult for people in walking and cycling programs to elevate their heart rate into the higher areas of their intensity prescription. They should be content to exceed the lower limit. This will be addressed again under duration.

DURATION

The second part of the program design is how long is a prolonged exercise session. How long do you have to exercise? Time requirements range from 20 to 60 minutes of exercise. The duration varies for different activity modes. The primary determining factor is the intensity level of the activity. If the intensity level is high, the duration can be reduced (jogging). If intensity is low, duration should be prolonged (walking). Another factor is whether the body weight is supported on the feet or by some equipment or water as with swimmers. Below is the recommended duration for some aerobic activities.

Activity Mode	Minimum Duration	Maximum Duration
Walking	30 Minutes	60 Minutes
Jogging	20 Minutes	40 Minutes
Swimming	30 Minutes	60 Minutes
Cycling	30 Minutes	60 Minutes
Aerobic Dance	20 Minutes	60 Minutes
Other Games	60 Minutes	

In swimming, the body weight is supported in part by the water that also contributes to cooling the body. In cycling, the body weight is supported by the cycle. Aerobic Dance routines vary with the difficulty and duration of each routine. Other games such as racquetball and basketball involve a good deal of starting and stopping, and therefore the duration must be extended.

Those who are starting out in an exercise program should favor the lower limit. At the beginning it may not be possible to maintain the activity for the minimum recommended time. Don't force yourself to the limit when starting out. It often takes some time to condition the muscular system to the point where it can sustain activity that will condition the cardiovascular system. It is also difficult to attain the upper levels of intensity limits in cycling and walking programs. In these modes of exercise, it is best to favor the lower intensity levels and upper duration levels. Research has shown that exercisers do not get a beneficial return on their time when they exceed the maximal limits. This applies to people who are exercising to gain physical fitness and not to those who are training for competition. Physical improvement can occur after the maximal time. This improvement is minimal, and for a recreational exerciser does not provide benefits equal to the time spent. For those exercising in preparation for a competitive event, the extra time spent training may provide the small improvement that separates first from second place.

FREQUENCY

The final factor in the design of the cardiovascular fitness program is how often must one exercise. The rule is three to five times per week. Again the beginner should be content with the lower level. A workout every other day will provide good conditioning and sufficient recovery between workouts. A lack of recovery time leaves one more susceptible to injuries. As one's level of fitness improves, the frequency of workouts can be increased. This will speed the conditioning process. It should be stressed that one must balance the desire for success and the risk of injury that can destroy all that has been achieved.

AEROBIC ACTIVITIES

The following are common activities used to develop cardiovascular endurance. Each requires specific technique to achieve maximum benefit. Proper technique and pacing methods are provided for each activity.

Walking

Many people do not view walking as an exercise mode. It may be that it is viewed as too easy and something that everyone can do. These may be the very reasons why walking is an excellent aerobic activity. Walking provides an activity with two distinct advantages. People who have been sedentary for long periods of time do not possess the muscular strength and endurance to participate in other vigorous physical activities without suffering muscle fatigue and much discomfort. In many cases the new exerciser must spend some time developing the strength and endurance of the leg muscle before they can start to stress the achievement of reaching aerobic intensity goals. Many people have selected walking as the form of exercise they prefer. They can achieve a very high level of aerobic fitness with this activity.

The proper technique for walking is to walk tall with your head up. Don't look down at your feet. Swing your arms in rhythm with your legs. The foot strike should be heel striking the ground first, rolling across the foot to push off the ball of the foot and the large toe.

The proper pace is determined by one's level of fitness. For those just starting out, a comfortable pace that allows them to achieve their time goal is best. As the leg muscles become stronger the pace can be increased. This is accomplished by lengthening the stride and swinging the arms with more gusto. Walkers will have difficulty raising the heart rate into the upper limits of the target heart rate zone. It is for this reason that the duration of a walking program must be increased. As conditioning improves the duration should range from 40 to 60 minutes.

Jogging

The jogging program requires from 20 to 40 minutes of exercise. Jogging is often listed as the best form of aerobic exercise because it has the shortest duration, requires little equipment and can be done individually virtually anywhere. The head should be carried high. Looking down at the feet causes a rounding of the back and poor posture. The arms should be carried at waist height. The shoulders should be relaxed. Don't clinch your fist. If this is a problem, place the thumb against the index finger as you run. The foot strike should be heel first, roll across the foot to push off the ball of the foot and the large toe. Let the ankle relax. The heel should strike the ground under the knee. This will prevent over striding and the slapping foot strike. Don't bounce and avoid extra body movement that detracts from the efficiency of the body.

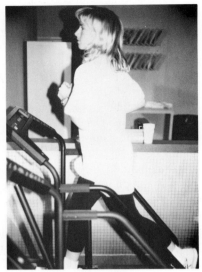

Figure 11-1

The most efficient method of pacing is the pulse check four to five minutes into the run. It is much easier to reach the median or upper limits of your heart rate range when jogging. It is for this reason that duration is less than when walking. With experience the talking method or perceive exertion can replace the pulse check.

Swimming

Aquatics provide an excellent mode for aerobic activity. Many assume that you must be able to swim to exercise in a pool. There are many activities that you can do. They include walking in water above your waist, bobbing in deeper water or doing a flutter kick at the side of the pool. Water aerobics is also a popular activity.

Aquatic exercise is an excellent activity mode since it involves all of the large muscle groups of the body. The resistance of the water provides not only for cardiovascular conditioning but also improves muscle conditioning.

Establishing the pace for swimming varies with the skill of the swimmer. The most common strokes used for exercise swimming are the crawl, sidestroke and elementary back stroke. The target heart rate sets the intensity limits for the program. For non swimmers doing exercise in the water, and the adjustment of the speed of these exercises provides for maintaining the proper intensity. Monitoring the pulse rate is easily accomplished.

Any swimmer can benefit from aquatics as a mode of exercise. A poor swimmer performs inefficiently and therefore wastes much effort, but this forces the pulse rate up to a higher intensity level that allows for a reduction in duration. This person may have to adapt an interval program such as swimming one length of the pool and then walking back to swim another. More accomplished swimmers may be able to adjust the intensity by changing strokes. This also helps to avoid muscle fatigue.

The advanced level swimmers will swim very efficiently. They may have difficulty raising their heart rate into the upper limits of the heart rate range. They can make adjustments for this by methods of restricting their speed with buoys and drag suits. Duration also can be extended.

Cycling

There are two forms of cycling that are used for cardiovascular exercise. Bicycling uses the traditional bike in an outdoor setting. Bicycling can be an excellent form of exercise. It requires the correct setting to achieve this goal. When using bicycling for exercise one must ride at a rapid pace, nonstop for a prolonged period of time. The difficulty is finding an area where this can be done without risk of injury to the exerciser.

The second method of cycling uses the indoor ergometer or stationary bike. This method delivers the same benefits as the outdoor style without the need for special areas and risk of injury. The difficulty is that many find this mode to be boring as they sit in the same place to do their exercise.

There are many bicycles and ergometers on the market. Bikes are constructed with light weight materials and are geared to adjust for hills and speed. Ergometers come in many forms with a wide variety of gadgets. Most of the gadgets do little for improving fitness but provide methods for monitoring heart rates, calories burned and motivation.

The primary technique in cycling is that the knee should be just slightly bent at the bottom of the pedal stroke. This provides for the most effective leg action.

Establishing the intensity of the cycling program again uses the target heart rate. One usually has to cycle more than twice as fast as they would run to attain a similar heart rate. It is often difficult to achieve the upper limits of the target range. For this reason the duration for cycling is usually extended to 30 to 60 minutes of exercise.

AEROBIC EXERCISES

This activity is often referred to as aerobic dance. It involves rhythmic movement using the arms and legs in routines of stepping, hopping and jumping in place. Usually these routines incorporate the use of recorded music. Often steps and mini tramps are used to provide variations to routines.

The major concern with this type of activity is the surface that it is performed on. Constant impact of the foot on a hard surface can result in injuries that will curtail participation. The target heart rate range provides the intensity level for the program. Periodic pulse checks will help to establish the appropriate pace. It is difficult to establish an activity duration level since intensity levels vary drastically from instructor to instructor. Lower levels equate to cycling while advanced levels are the equivalent of jogging.

OTHER EQUIPMENT

Other indoor exercise equipment includes rowers, stairclimbers and treadmills. Each can provide excellent cardiovascular exercise.

Treadmills provide an indoor setting for walking/jogging programs. They allow for establishing the speed desired and the terrain with elevation adjustments. Most treadmills provide side rails for maintaining one's balance. When one becomes accustomed to the treadmill, they should try to avoid supporting their weight with their hands on the side rails. Supporting your weight in this manner substantially reduces the workload encountered.

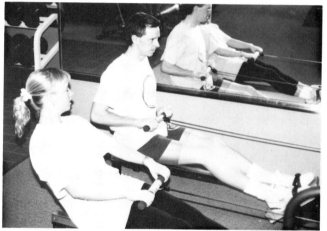

Rowers provide a form of cardiovascular exercise that uses both the upper and lower body. Proper technique requires the use of the legs to push to a straight leg position and the pulling with the arms to complete the stroke.

Stairclimbers use a common task that is among the most difficult that we encounter. When walking up stairs one has to lift their body weight against the force of gravity.

Proper technique requires the exerciser to maintain an upright position. The side rails are provided for balance. Avoid supporting your weight on the side rails with your arms. This reduces the weight that your legs are lifting thus making the task easier and benefits less.

Figure 11-2

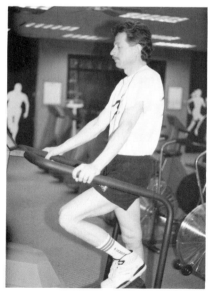

Figure 11-3

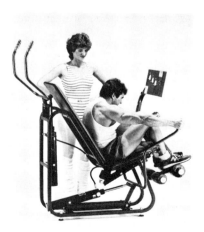

Figure 11-4

PHYSIOLOGICAL CHANGES

Regular exercise places increased demands upon the body's systems. In the case of aerobic exercise these demands are placed upon the cardiovascular system. As a result of these demands, the cardiovascular system changes to better meet these physical demands. The following are specific changes that occur with regular cardiovascular training.

PULMONARY FUNCTION

The muscles of the respiratory system become stronger. This provides for more air to be moved into the lungs. Vital capacity is a genetic endowment, but sedentary people usually function at less than optimal capacity. Swimmers have documented this capability to provide more complete filling of the lungs thus making more oxygen available for energy production.

CIRCULATORY SYSTEM

There is some evidence of increased blood vessel size and collateral circulation. These changes make the diffusion of blood and oxygen to the tissues much greater. Also regular exercise causes an increase in blood volume and an increase in hemoglobin. These changes provide the vehicle for the transportation of more oxygen to the tissues.

HEART FUNCTION

The heart muscle increases in strength and size with regular aerobic exercise. Enhanced myocardial contractility results in greater emptying of the left ventricle. This results in the capability of pumping greater volumes of blood into the arterial system. Greater blood volumes mean greater availability of oxygen to the cells. The physiological changes resulting from aerobic exercise are:

1. Increased stroke volume.
2. Decreased resting and exercise heart rates.
3. Reduced oxygen demand by the heart muscle because of the reduced heart rate.
4. Increased collateral circulation that increases oxygen diffusion to the heart muscle.

ENERGY PRODUCTION

Additional oxygen supplies are of no value unless they can be used in the production of energy. There are several physiological changes that provide for greater oxygen utilization and therefore greater energy production. Some of these follow.

1. An increase in the number, size and membrane surface of mitrochondria. These are the "power plants" of energy production that contain the enzymes needed for energy transformation.
2. An increase in the enzymes responsible for the creation of aerobic energy in the muscles.
3. Increases in resting levels of anaerobic substrate that increases potential anaerobic capacity.
4. Skeletal muscle myoglobin content increases. The result is an increase in the amount of oxygen within the cell at anyone time.
5. An increase in the trained muscles ability to mobilize and oxidize fat.
6. The trained muscle has a greater capacity to oxidize carbohydrates.

WASTE REMOVAL

The improved capacity to circulate blood provides for the more efficient removal of the wastes of oxidation. Carbon dioxide and lactic acid are removed from the muscle cells. Heat is a major by product of exercise. Heat is moved from the tissue level to the surface of the body where it can be dissipated into the atmosphere. The trained body can work better in hot climates, since it is able to dissipate heat more readily. Thus the body can better cool itself.

CARDIOVASCULAR DISEASE RISK REDUCTION

There is no documented cause of cardiovascular disease. The following conditions have been associated with the disease. Persons with these conditions have an increased risk of cardiovascular disease. These conditions are called risk factors. There are two categories of risk factors. The unchangeable risk factors are the ones that you cannot control. They include:

1. Positive family history
2. Advanced age

3. Male sex
4. Race

The changeable risk factors are the ones that you can control. They include:

1. Hypertension
2. Hyperlipidemia
   a. Triglycerides
   b. Cholesterol
3. Cigarette smoking
4. Obesity
5. Psychological or emotional distress
6. Glucose intolerance
7. Physical inactivity

One's risk of cardiovascular disease can be reduced drastically as the result of regular aerobic exercise. It has been shown that regular aerobic exercise has a positive impact on some changeable risk factors.

Many people with moderately elevated blood pressure have seen reductions as the result of exercise.

Increases in high density lipoprotein (HDL) cholesterol has occurred when people do aerobic exercise. HDL cholesterol helps to move fats through the blood stream. The increase in HDL improves the ratio of total cholesterol.

Cigarette smokers who adhere to a regular aerobic exercise programs have a high smoking cessation rate. This is not true for other game types of recreational activities.

Regular physical activity may be the best long range method of weight reduction. It has been documented that weight loss programs that do not include exercise result in muscle and fat loses. Weight loss, as a result of exercise, is a slow process. The extended lifestyle change can help the weight loss to become permanent.

The psychological benefits are numerous. They include bolstered self image, more self confidence, better sleep, ability to cope with stress and eased depression.

These all tend to revolve around liking oneself more. When you like yourself, your rate of success in all tasks that you do often increases.

Regular physical exercise enhances the transport of blood glucose. This means that diabetics may become somewhat less dependent upon insulin.

There are eleven risk factors associated with cardiovascular disease. Four are beyond individual control. On the other hand, the changeable risk factors respond positively to regular physical exercise. Thus it can be said that aerobic exercise can help to save your life. For many years we have known that physical exercise can improve the quality of life. Recently however, Dr. Ralph Paffenbarger and Dr. Kenneth Cooper have shown through documented studies that physical exercise also can increase the quantity of life.

Physical exercise is hard work. But it can help you to enjoy life more and live longer. Look for an appealing activity and get started today. It is never too early or too late to begin.

SUMMARY

To enter an aerobic fitness program successfully, one must identify the proper intensity and duration for their program. Frequency and mode are the other two important design factors. Proper technique is important if the desired workout is to be achieved. The nature of some activities reduces the intensity level thus requiring an increase in the duration of the activity. Through the physiological changes from exercise, the human body is able to get more air into the body. It has the capacity to transport more oxygen through the vascular system. It also increases the ability to circulate oxygen rich blood due to a stronger heart muscle. With a greater oxygen supply available, the body takes advantage of the situation by improving it's ability to produce energy. A concluding capability is the improved ability to remove the wastes of oxidation. Thus it has been shown that regular aerobic exercise changes the human body to make it a more effective machine.

Name _____ Grade _____

WORKSHEET 11-A

Chapter Eleven—Aerobic Training Principles

Matching: Put the letter of the definition next to the word/phrase.

Words/Phrases

1. Mode
2. Intensity
3. Time
4. Frequency
5. Jogging
6. Walking
7. Cross Country Skiing
8. Cycling
9. 220
10. 220–age
11. 90%
12. 60%
13. Pulse Check
14. 60 minutes
15. 20 minutes
16. Five days a week
17. Three days a week
18. Treadmills
19. Cycle ergometers
20. Rowers
21. Stairclimbers
22. Heart strength
23. More blood pumped
24. More oxygen available
25. Risk factor reduction
26. Hypertension lowered
27. Hyperlipidemia lowered
28. Smoking cessation
29. Obesity
30. Glucose intolerance

1. _____
2. _____
3. _____
4. _____
5. _____
6. _____
7. _____
8. _____
9. _____
10. _____
11. _____
12. _____
13. _____
14. _____
15. _____
16. _____
17. _____
18. _____
19. _____
20. _____
21. _____
22. _____
23. _____
24. _____
25. _____
26. _____
27. _____
28. _____
29. _____
30. _____

Definitions

A. Cardiovascular risk factor reduced by regular exercise.
B. Cardiovascular risk factor reduced by regular exercise.
C. General outcome of regular exercise.
D. Physiological improvement of heart function through regular exercise.
E. Aerobic exercise equipment.
F. Aerobic exercise equipment.

G.   Minimum number of days recommended for exercise per week.

H.   Minimum recommended length of an exercise bout in minutes.

I.   Method of monitoring the intensity level of exercise.

J.   Recommended maximum intensity level of exercise.

K.   Theoretical maximum for human heart beats per minute.

L.   A mode of aerobic exercise.

M.   A mode of aerobic exercise.

N.   Criteria for length of an exercise bout.

O.   Type of exercise being done.

P.   Cardiovascular disease risk factor reduced by regular exercise.

Q.   Cardiovascular disease risk factor reduced by regular exercise.

R.   Cardiovascular disease risk factor reduced by regular exercise.

S.   Physiological benefit of regular exercise.

T.   Physiological benefit of regular exercise.

U.   Aerobic exercise equipment.

V.   Aerobic exercise equipment.

W.   Recommended maximum number of exercise days per week.

X.   Recommended maximum length in minutes of an exercise bout.

Y.   Minimum level of intensity of exercise.

Z.   How to obtain your age adjusted maximum heart rate.

AA.   Mode of aerobic exercise.

BB.   Mode of aerobic exercise.

CC.   Criteria for how often one should exercise.

DD.   Criteria for how hard one should exercise.

CHAPTER TWELVE
Training Principles

PRETEST—POSTEST

In order to determine the effectiveness of a training program or simply to monitor change, it is a recommended practice to gather data before and after the program. This is called the "pretest-postest" concept. (Use worksheet 12 A, located at the end of this chapter to record personal data).

The data that is gathered is specific to the components of the program. In other words, exercises that are part of the program will be tested before and after. In strength programs, the person should be pretested on the apparatus that he/she is going to use during the program. (Ex. Free Wt. training program—test using Free Wts.) Also the person should have adequate practice to ensure that they are familiar with the exercise and the piece of equipment being used. This will all contribute to the validity and reliability of the data.

TESTING METHODS—TYPES OF RESISTANCES

The most common and simplest method of testing for strength is called the **1 RM (One Repetition Maximum)**. The person being tested identifies the maximum amount of weight that he/she can move one time through a complete range of motion using the trial and error method. The person will lift gradually increasing weight until the point of failure is reached. The last successful repetition is then recorded as the 1 RM for that particular exercise.

The 1 RM method would be an example of an **isotonic** resistance, which is a fixed resistance that doesn't change as the lever moves. Free weights and weight stack equipment are examples of isotonic resistances and are gravity based. Most isotonic resistances are gravity based with the exception of the Keiser equipment which uses air pressure as its resistance.

Another method is called **isometric** where there is no movement at all. The resistance is greater than any force the person might be able to apply. A hand grip dynamometer is an example of that type.

Hydraulic equipment uses a lever that is connected to a hydraulic cylinder that contains a fixed amount of oil. By applying force or torque to the lever, the person is trying to push a fixed amount of oil through a fixed size opening. The force that is applied creates pressure within the cylinder and that pressure is then measured by a gauge. HydraFitness equipment uses hydraulic resistance.

Regardless of the type of equipment used, certain basic training principles need to be adhered to in order to ensure a safe and effective program. Whether a person uses free weights, weight stacks, hydraulics or pneumatics, these basic principles should be applied.

The following is a presentation of these important principles.

SYMMETRY

Both sides of the body need to be trained the same. The body is anatomically symmetrical. That is, the human body has the same muscles and bones on one side as it has on the other. And to ensure that both sides are developed equally, they both need to be trained equally. Unilateral work (working each side independent of the other, as in dumbbells) makes each side of the body to do its own work. Bilateral work (single levers like barbells) doesn't isolate the sides, which means that a stronger side would do more work than a weaker side. Work done is directly correlated to training improvement. Therefore whenever possible, unilateral work is recommended.

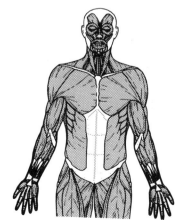

Figure 12-1. Symmetry

BALANCE

Muscles are arranged in opposing pairs that have opposite actions. The quad/ham pair is a good example (See Figure 12-2). The quadricep, located on the front of the thigh, straightens the knee. The hamstring, located on the back of the thigh, bends the knee. The relationship between the two is called muscle balance. Ideally these two muscle groups should be equal in strength, but in reality they aren't. This is called muscle imbalance. Muscle imbalance can occur incidental to normal movement because one pair is required to do more work, such as the quadricep having to propulse the body with the hamstring only having to lift the lower leg. Or it can occur through poorly designed and executed training programs when only one of the pairs is trained, and the other is neglected. Biomechanically, one of the pairs is the accelerator for human movement, and the other is the brake. In order to ensure safe and effective movement, both pairs should be trained equally.

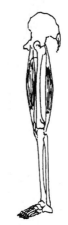

Figure 12-2 Balance

ISOLATION

Improvement in muscle performance is directly related to the work that it is required to do. Therefore it is much more efficient to target a specific muscle to do the work, while simultaneously limiting the effect of secondary or unwanted movement. This principle is called isolation. Figure 12-3 shows a free weight bicep curl being done with the should blades pinned to the wall. This position will eliminate the unwanted movements of hip and shoulder sway which could assist the bicep in the action. Failure to limit movement will result in poor efficiency and inaccurate feedback. The user thinks he/she can lift a certain weight when in fact, if isolated he/she would not be able to do it.

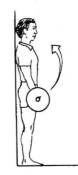

Figure 12-3 Isolated Curl

RANGE OF MOTION

Strength gains occur only at the angle at which the muscle is trained. In order to ensure that strength gains occur throughout the full range of motion, the user must go through the full range of motion on every rep. Figure 12-4 shows this principle. "X" is the shoulder, "Y" is the elbow, and "Z" is the hand. In a properly executed curling action, the hand should start at position "A" and complete the entire arc by finishing at position "B". Done improperly, which is often the case with the bicep curl, the hand starts at "C" and finishes at "D" completing a short arc. During the first rep, the muscle is stressed through the complete range of motion which means training occurred at all angles. In the second short arc rep, training will only occur in the shaded areas.

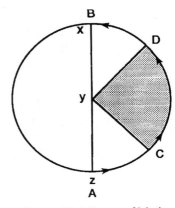

Figure 12-4 Range of Motion

OVERLOAD

In order for strength gains to occur, the resistance on the muscle must be overload, which is defined as 60% of current maximum. Exercising against a resistance that is not an overload would be a form of endurance not strength training. It is essential then that an overload be identified, so that an accurate exercise prescription can be made. Furthermore as training progresses, resistances must be increased to ensure that the overload continues. Muscles get stronger, which means that current resistances could fall below overload thresholds resulting in strength gains plateauing.

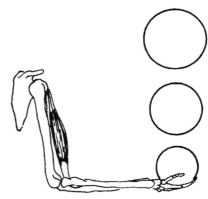

Figure 12-5 Overload

Joint Mechanics

The potential for the human body to apply force (straight line action) or torque (action around a fixed point) varies according to the joint angle. This is due to the mechanics of the human lever system. Figure 12-6 shows the angles and the relative torque of those angles. The human body is strongest at 90 degrees and weakest at 180. The human lever system also loses strength in both directions as it progresses away from 90 degrees. The implication is that the most effective programs will have varying resistances to accommodate the lever system principles.

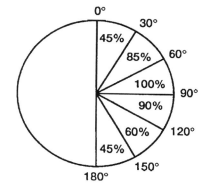

Figure 12-6 Lever System Torque Angles

Respiration

The body cannot store oxygen. It must have a continuous and adequate resupply in order for the cells to carry on their vital functions. The only source of oxygen is a regular respiration rate, which when interrupted causes a reduction of oxygen flow to the cells. When the cells, in this case the muscle cells, do not receive an adequate supply, their functioning is impaired. This can occur in a number of ways. Withholding oxygen by holding one's breath, or working at a level of intensity that exceeds the body's oxygen delivery capacity are two examples. They both create an anaerobic condition, which by nature is time limited.

The implication for the exerciser is that holding one's breath is in fact withholding the fuel that the muscles need to do the work. It is basically counterproductive to what they are trying to do. The exerciser should breathe at a rate that is determined by the level of intensity of the work being done. The higher the work level the higher the respiration rate should be.

The exerciser should never use the "Valsalva Maneuver" during the work. It is best described as a forced false expiration, which manifests itself as a "grunt". This is a particularly dangerous habit that can actually inhibit chest cavity blood flow. The best recommendation is that the "inspiration" breath should be held very briefly just prior to initiating the rep. But once the movement has begun (moment of inertia), the expiration should begin immediately. The inspiration just prior to the movement helps to stabilize the chest vertebrae and is recommended. However, expiration should begin immediately after movement to dissipate the chest pressures so as not to adversely impact blood flow to the heart.

Alternative Days

The rule for exercise frequency is simply that the length of the restorative phase is determined by the level of the intensity of the workout bout. If a person works out very hard one day, he/she should not do the same thing the next day. There should be at least one days rest in between in order to give the body a chance to repair/restore itself prior to the next hard workout. A high intensity workout is defined as a overload which is 60% of current maximum.

Working out the same way at the same high level of intensity on consecutive days will eventually become counterproductive. Performance will go down and injury frequency will go up.

If daily exercise is required or desired, the exercise prescriptions should be different. An example would be to weight train one day and do an aerobic workout the next. Or if the same type of workout is desired, vary the body parts involved. Example would be to weight train the upper body one day and the lower body the next.

For low intensity workouts, there is no extended time needed for restoration. These kinds of workouts can be done on consecutive days without the concern for an increase in injury frequency. However boredom can be a problem, so variety is recommended here also.

Name _____ Date _____

WORKSHEET 12–A

Keiser 1 RM Scoresheet

STRENGTH SCORES

1. LOWER BACK   Pre_____   Post_____

2. RIGHT ARM CURL   Pre_____   Post_____

3. LEFT ARM CURL.   Pre_____   Post_____

4. RIGHT TRICEP   Pre_____   Post_____

5. LEFT TRICEP   Pre_____   Post_____

6. LAT. SH. RAISE   Pre_____   Post_____

7. MILITARY PRESS   Pre_____   Post_____

8. SEATED CHEST PR.   Pre_____   Post_____

9. SEATED BUTTERFLY   Pre_____   Post_____

10. LAT PULL   Pre_____   Post_____

11. UPPER BACK   Pre_____   Post_____

12. ABDOMINAL   Pre_____   Post_____

13. SQUAT   Pre_____   Post_____

14. RIGHT LEG PRESS   Pre_____   Post_____

15. LEFT LEG PRESS   Pre_____   Post_____

16. RIGHT LEG CURL   Pre_____   Post_____

17. LEFT LEG CURL   Pre_____   Post_____

18. RT. LEG EXT.   Pre_____   Post_____

19. L. LEG EXT.   Pre_____   Post_____

20. HIP ADDUCTION   Pre_____   Post_____

21. HIP ABDUCTION   Pre_____   Post_____

WORKSHEET 12-B

Chapter Twelve—Training Principles

1. Skeletal muscle is arranged anatomically symmetrical.   1._____

2. Functionally, skeletal muscle is symmetrical.   2._____

3. Unilateral training is not recommended.   3._____

4. Work done by the muscle is directly correlated to the training effect.   4._____

5. Muscles arranged in opposition is called balance.   5._____

6. Functionally, imbalance does not exist in the human.   6._____

7. A common error is to train only one pair.   7._____

8. Opposing pairs have a brake and accelerator relationship.   8._____

9. Isolation improves exercise efficiency.   9._____

10. Poor isolation does not effect the accuracy of the feedback.   10._____

11. Strength gains occur specific to the joint angle trained.   11._____

12. Short arc training is a common error.   12._____

13. Overload is defined as 40% of current maximum strength.   13._____

14. It is not necessary to train with an overload to ensure strength gains.   14._____

15. Pretesting helps to determine the appropriate exercise prescriptions.   15._____

16. The human body is strongest at 180 degree angles.   16._____

17. The human body is weakest at 90 degree angles.   17._____

18. A fixed resistance accommodates the lever system.   18._____

19. The body can store oxygen.   19._____

20. The only source of oxygen is regular respiration.   20._____

21. Withholding oxygen is a common training error.   21._____

22. Anaerobic exercise is not time limited.   22._____

23. The respiration rate should be determined by the level of exercise intensity.   23._____

24. The Valsalva maneuver is a recommended exercise practice.   24._____

25. The weight trainer should exhale during exertion.   25._____

26. The length of the restorative phase is determined by the level of intensity of work.   26._____

27. The same muscles should be worked at high intensity on consecutive days.   27._____

28. Aerobic and anaerobic exercise can be alternated if daily exercise is desired.   28._____

29. Inadequate rest can result in over use injuries.   29._____

30. Low intensity work can be done safely on consecutive days.   30._____

Name _____ Date _____

WORKSHEET 12–C

Paramount 1 RM Scoresheet

1. PULLOVER   Pre_____   Post_____

2. SEATED CHEST PRESS   Pre_____   Post_____

3. VERTICAL BUTTERFLY   Pre_____   Post_____

4. DELTOID   Pre_____   Post_____

5. SHOULDER PRESS   Pre_____   Post_____

6. TRICEP EXTENSION   Pre_____   Post_____

7. BICEP CURL   Pre_____   Post_____

8. ABDOMINALS   Pre_____   Post_____

9. LOWER BACK   Pre_____   Post_____

10. LEG CURL   Pre_____   Post_____

11. LEG EXTENSION   Pre_____   Post_____

12. OUTER THIGH   Pre_____   Post_____

13. INNER THIGH   Pre_____   Post_____

14. ROTARY TORSO R   Pre_____   Post_____

15. ROTARY TORSO L   Pre_____   Post_____

16. LAT. PULL   Pre_____   Post_____

CHAPTER THIRTEEN
Weight Training Principles

The focus of this chapter will be to prepare the individual to design and develop a weight training program. The most important step in designing a weight training program is to determine what the person desires as an outcome. This chapter will address weight training programs, specific muscle types, types of strength exercises, various weight training equipment, purposes and principles of weight training, and safety measures.

MUSCLE TYPES

Weight training is a form of exercise that is designed to increase the strength and/or endurance of muscle tissue. The human body is composed of three types of muscle tissue: smooth, cardiac and skeletal.

Smooth Muscle Tissue

This muscle tissue is involuntary and lines the hollow organs of the body. Blood vessels and the intestines are examples of organs whose walls are composed of smooth muscle. Weight training does not effect smooth muscle tissue.

Cardiac Muscle Tissue

This muscle tissue is found only in the heart. It can be strengthened by exercise. Aerobic exercise that is rhythmic with a prolonged duration is the most common method used to condition cardiac muscle. Weight training can strengthen cardiac muscle if circuit training is used with no rest between stations. Weight training is not the normal method used to strengthen cardiac muscle. The strenuous nature of weight training without rest reduces the adherence to the program.

Skeletal (Striated) Muscle Tissue

The human body has over 600 skeletal muscles that work to provide human movement. This muscle tissue is the primary type of muscle fiber that is developed by weight training.

Skeletal muscle has two distinct types of fibers. Red (slow twitch) fibers are better suited for endurance/aerobic activities. White (fast twitch) fibers are better suited for explosive activities of short duration.

Muscle fibers function under the all-or-none principle. This means that when the muscle fibers contract, all of the muscle fibers of the motor unit will contract completely or not at all. The brain will determine the anticipated force required to complete a given job. It will than recruit, through the nervous system, the appropriate number of motor units needed to complete the job.

TYPES OF STRENGTH EXERCISE

There are three types of exercise that are used to develop muscular strength, endurance and power. Each varies due to the movement and resistance.

Isometric

Isometric exercise is when the contraction of the muscle group does not cause movement of the resistance. The fibers are contracting and yet no movement occurs at the joint. The resistance is an immovable object. The resistance is equal or greater than the force exerted.

Isotonic

Isotonic exercise occurs when the muscle contracts through the range of motion causing the resistance to move through space. The resistance can be any object where the resistance remains constant throughout the range of motion. Free weights are an example of isotonic exercise.

Isokinetic

Isokinetic exercise is similar to isotonic exercise in that the resistance is moved. It differs in that the resistance from weights is accommodated to the strengths and weaknesses of the individual muscle. The machine controls the speed, velocity and resistance throughout the range of motion. Weight stack machines are an example.

TYPES OF WEIGHT TRAINING EQUIPMENT

Calisthenics

The simplest form of weight training does not require expensive equipment. It uses the individual's body weight as the resistance. Push-ups, sit-ups, chin-ups and dips are examples of weight training exercises that can be done without equipment. This form of training can yield equal results to that of expensive equipment forms.

Free Weights

This form of weight training equipment uses barbells and dumbbells. Training programs utilizing free weights are varied, and the design of individual programs will be based upon individual goals. Free weights require more commitment, both in the length of individual workouts and the number of days involved. The nature of free weight training provides for movement in any plane and therefore the number of lifts is countless.

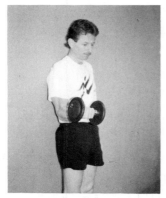

Figure 13-1

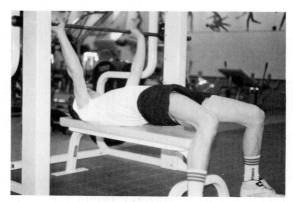

Figure 13-2

Weight Stacks

This form of weight training involves the use of stacks of weight plates that are connected via a cable or chain. The individual selects the amount of weight to be used by inserting a pin in the stack of plates. The weight stacks can only be moved in the planes defined by the machine. This limits the number of lifts that can be used in muscle development. Cybex and Paramount are two brand names of weight stack equipment.

Air Pressure

Keiser is a brand name that uses air pressure as the form of resistance. An air compressor produces air pressure that is fed to each machine via a connecting hose. The person weight training adjusts the resistance by increasing or decreasing the amount of air pressure. In performance it is similar to weight stacks.

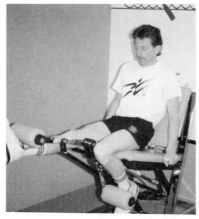

Figure 13-3

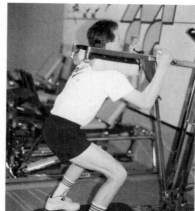

Figure 13-4

Hydraulics

Hydrafitness equipment uses hydraulic fluid in hydraulic cylinders as the resistance. These machines, like Keiser and weight stacks, limit movement to the planes established by the machine. Hydrafitness has the advantage of doing flexion and extension exercises on one piece of equipment. Weight stacks and air pressure machines require two separate machines to do the same workout.

PURPOSES FOR WEIGHT TRAINING

There are five basic programs that utilize weight training. An individual must determine their purpose before formatting a program of exercise.

Power Lifting

Power lifting is a competitive event where. The lifters compete by weight class in three standard lifts. These include:

1. Bench Press
2. Squat
3. Dead Lift

Olympic Lifting

Olympic lifting is another form of competitive weight lifting. Olympic lifting is conducted at regional, national and international events. Competition is in two lifts, the clean and jerk and the snatch. Competitors compete in weight classes with the winners determined by the total amount of weight successfully lifted.

Body Builders

Body Building is another form of competition that utilizes weight training as a preparation tool. Body builders spend countless hours working on development of size, cut and definition of the muscular system.

Weight Trainers

The classification of weight trainers identifies individuals who are lifting to develop muscular strength, endurance or power for the express purpose of performing a task more efficiently. These people include athletes or persons who wish to tone the muscular system to make any physical tasks easier to perform.

Principles of Weight Training

The F.I.T. program is a method of designing a safe, effective workout program using the following guidelines. F.I.T. means:

1. Frequency or how often the program must be implemented. A minimum of three times per week is required with free weight programs often requiring more workouts.
2. Intensity is a measurement of the workload. The workload or resistance is based upon the number of Reps and Sets that are required. Reps refers to the number of times the weight is lifted. Sets are groups of Reps. An example would be a program calling for three Sets of 50 Reps of abdominal crunches. Each Set requires that 50 crunches be performed before rest can occur.
3. Time is the length of the exercise session. Weight training is designed around Reps and Sets and not a time frame as in Aerobic exercise. With weight stack types of equipment, that provide for easy weight adjustment, a program can be completed in the 30 minute range. Free weights may take up to two hours for a complete workout.

BREATHING

When one exerts force in weight training a common fault is holding their breath. This is a very dangerous practice. The breathing technique should follow this simple rule exhale during the greatest exertion (the lift phase) and inhale when lowering the weight.

OVERLOAD

The overload principle is the best method to use when training to increase muscular strength. The overload is accomplished by training with at least 60 percent of the 1 Rm and attempting more repetitions. As the load is changed the resistance should slowly be increased to insure that injuries will not occur in the muscle groups being trained.

PROGRESSIVE RESISTANCE

Weight training is a form of progressive exercise where the resistance is slowly increased as the body accommodates to the resistance that is applied. The goal of progressive resistance exercise is to do between 5 - 8 Reps in Sets of 1 - 5. When the maximum goal for Reps and Sets is achieved, the resistance should be increased. It is important to remember that the lower extremities and torso can lift more and be trained at greater levels. Increases in resistance should be made at ten pound increments for the lower body and five pound increments for the upper body.

SPECIFICITY

The principle of specificity states that the training program must specifically exercise the muscles that you are trying to develop (either for power, sport or fitness). In other words, if the individual is attempting to increase speed they would lift light weights and do high speed repetitions. Their strength program should closely resemble the activity that they are training for.

CIRCUIT TRAINING

This is a form of weight training that makes use of multiple stations. Usually these circuits involve performing activity on weight training machines using moderate weight, and the goal is 8 - 12 Reps at each station. The individual moves directly from one station to the next without rest periods between stations.

NEGATIVES

Negatives are used to describe the ability of the muscle to lower a weight, even though the individual is unable to lift the weight. Use of negatives occur when your training partner raises the weight for you when you have hit failure. You would then lower the weight and then repeat the procedure until you are no longer able to do so. Negative workouts are an advanced technique that should not be used by beginners.

PERIODIZATION (TRAINING CYCLES)

Periodization is an advanced training technique where the individual increases the intensity toward a predetermined peak. Then after achieving the goal, backs off using lighter weights for a break and then begins the cycle again.

PYRAMID TRAINING

This is a training system that involves the use of multiple Sets, where the first Set is performed with light resistance (50% of 1RM), and the goal is 10 - 15 Reps. This is a warm up Set. The second set is done with greater resistance (75% of I RM) with fewer Reps attempted. The last Set is done at heavy resistance (greater than 90% of I RM) and 2 - 5 Reps are attempted. A pyramid program can be pyramided up, up and down or just down. By incorporating different approaches the program will not get stale and interest and results will improve.

WEIGHT TRAINING WORKOUT DESIGN

Warm-up

Always start your program with a ten minute warm-up period. This should include warm-up activities as well as stretching exercises.

Weight Training Program

The weight training workout will involve reps and sets with predetermined resistances. The following conditions will control the actual design of the program:

1. Type of weight training equipment to be used.
2. Amount of time available.
3. Goal of the program: muscular strength, muscular endurance, or power.

Frequency of Workouts

The most accepted method for weight training involves workouts on alternate days. The rule is not to train a muscle group on consecutive days. This provides for rest and recovery for the muscles that are strenuously used. Often intense weight trainers will work out every day. They can do this without suffering injuries by training different muscles groups each day.

Weight Increases

When the individual achieves his/her goal for reps and sets, the resistance must be increased in accordance with the progressive resistance principle. The accepted rule is ten percent increases for lower extremities and torso and five percent increases for the upper body.

Log

People who exercise have found that a very good motivator is the maintenance of a training log. This is especially useful in weight training. Reps, sets and resistance should be recorded. This enables the exerciser to keep track of the progress and to know what work has to be done each day.

Spotter

It is very important when using free weights to have a workout partner. The partner can offer encouragement but they also provide assistance when failure is imminent, providing for a safe workout. Many weight trainers, working alone, have been injured when fatigue sets in and heavy weights cannot be safely managed.

Pain

Pain is a message from the body that something is wrong. If you suffer pain or are not feeling well STOP immediately. Do not resume your workout until you are feeling better.

Clothing

Always exercise in comfortable clothing that allows complete freedom of movement. Always wear shoes and when lifting free weights a weight belt is mandatory.

Cool Down

When you have completed your weight training program, you should finish up with a cool down program. This often is a repeat of the warm-up routine in reverse.

WORKSHEET 13-A

Chapter Thirteen—Weight Training Principles

Matching: Put the letter of the definition next to the word/phrase.

Words/Phrases

1.	Weight Training	1. _____
2.	Smooth Muscle	2. _____
3.	Cardiac Muscle	3. _____
4.	Skeletal Muscle	4. _____
5.	Isometric Exercise	5. _____
6.	Isotonic Exercise	6. _____
7.	Isokinetic Exercise	7. _____
8.	Calisthenics	8. _____
9.	Free Weights	9. _____
10.	Weight Stacks	10. _____
11.	Air Pressure	11. _____
12.	Hydraulics	12. _____
13.	Power Lifting	13. _____
14.	Olympic Lifting	14. _____
15.	Body Building	15. _____
16.	Overload Principle	16. _____
17.	Progressive Resistance	17. _____
18.	Isolation	18. _____
19.	Circuit Training	19. _____
20.	Negatives	20. _____
21.	Periodization	21. _____
22.	Reps	22. _____
23.	Sets	23. _____
24.	Resistance	24. _____
25.	Pyramid Training	25. _____

Definitions

A. Multiple sets with increasing amount of work per set—low to high.

B. Grouping of reps.

C. Varying the degree of workload during the training cycle.

D. Use of multiple stations, each for specific exercise.

E. Gradually increasing the workload during the training cycle.

F. Form of competition to determine physique development.

G. Form of competition to determine who can lift the most weight in 3 standard lifts.

H. Form of resistance used in some training equipment.

I. Form of resistance using gravity based dumbbells and barbells.

J. Exercise against a speed set resistance machine.

K. Exercise against an immovable resistance.

L. Muscle found only in the heart.

M. Form of training using resistance to develop skeletal muscle.

N. Force encountered by the muscle during exercise.

O. Number of times an exercise is repeated.

P. Resisting the force as the muscle extends.

Q. Targeting the muscle for specific work while limiting other muscle influence.

R. Giving the muscle more work to do than its done before.

S. Form of competition to determine maximum weight lifted in two standard lifts.

T. Machines using a fluid based resistance.

U. Machines using gravity arranged in a pulley plate system.

V. Endurance exercise using the gravity of the body as a resistance.

W. Exercise against a fixed resistance.

X. Muscle that moves the skeleton.

Y. Involuntary muscle found in the vital organs.

CHAPTER FOURTEEN
Ergogenic Aids

The many benefits of being active have become apparent to those who have adopted an active healthy lifestyle. However, some are not completely satisfied with their results. They want more, and as with any activity (school, work, relationships) that requires commitment. There are those that truly desire a short cut. Some are willing to try "magical" pills that guarantee weight loss overnight. Others are willing to try liposuction to remove excess fat cells, and others are willing to use passive weight machines that perform the activity for them.

This chapter will focus on those individuals who are looking for the short cuts, the quick and easy results. Specifically, those who want to be bigger, stronger, faster and more aggressive magically. The discussion in this chapter will focus on the use of ergogenic aids. Ergogenic Aids are those drugs/substances that are used for the enhancement or improvement of physical performance. For the majority of us, ergogenic aids would never be considered, although some everyday substances (such as caffeine) are classified as ergogenic aids. Usage problems of ergogenic aids are more widely seen at the competitive level, from the high school athlete to the elite Olympic or professional level. This chapter will examine the common ergogenic aids, how they effect the body and the positive and negative outcomes from such usage.

The reported benefits are varied for ergogenic aids, but the following list are some of the major reported effects of ergogenic aids.

1. There is an increase in muscular strength, size and power.
2. There is an increase in aggressive behavior.
3. The usage of ergogenic aids is beneficial in controlling weight loss.
4. There will be an increase in speed and acceleration.
5. That eye/hand coordination will increase.
6. They help relax the individual, thereby reducing stress.
7. Concentration will increase with usage.
8. Increase in competitive attitude of the user.
9. The user will have a lower pain perception.
10. The user will experience an increase in endurance.

Remember that these are potential outcomes. The research is not conclusive as to the actual benefits of all ergogenic aids. As with any drug use, the potential benefits are often negated by the potential negative side effects. There are countless articles dealing with the cost of ergogenic aid use. Len Bias was drafted by the Boston Celtics and died from cocaine use shortly after the draft. Ben Johnson, Gold Medal Winner, who tested positive for steroids and was stripped of the medal. Brian Bozworth was banned from the Orange Bowl Game after he tested positive for steroid usage. He was later drafted and played professional football, but his career was cut short due to injury (possibly related to his steroid use).

Lyle Alzado died after a successful professional football career. He contributed his early death to his continued use of anabolic steroids during his career. These are but a few of the many stories about negative consequences from ergogenic aid usage. The following is a list of the potential negative outcomes.

1. Impairment of judgement, reaction time, coordination, and balance. These are the main categories of skill, and these negative effects will obviously effect the athlete.
2. Eye-hand coordination is greatly reduced.
3. The muscular system of the body is damaged, reducing strength, flexibility, and increasing the potential for injury in sport and fitness pursuits.

4. Over-aggressive behavior, where the individual loses control and becomes violent for no apparent reason. With steroid use, this violent behavior has been given the name "roid rage". Other negative side-effects of steroid use will be discussed later in this chapter.

Obviously the negative side-effects are significant, yet the question still remains as to why the continued widespread use and growth of ergogenic usage in this country and the world. The answers are many: an average athlete trying to make the team, a way to reduce the pressure of athletics/life, a weight lifter who wants to be stronger and larger, or someone who wants to gain an edge against the competition. Whatever the reasons, usage is continually growing and no end is in sight. A better educational program in the school and for the parents is the only way to stem the tide of individuals who are willing to try any short cuts to improve their performance.

DIFFERENT TYPES OF ERGOGENIC AIDS

Caffeine—is one of the most commonly used ergogenic aids that has a long history of use and abuse, especially among endurance athletes and college students. Within the body, caffeine acts as a stimulant. Although most Americans don't think of caffeine as an ergogenic aid, it does appear on the list of banned substances by the International Olympic Committee (IOC). Although to reach the limits set by the IOC you would have to drink 6-8 cups of coffee (or other caffeine drinks) within several hours of the test.

Caffeine is found in many popular foods and is therefore a stimulant that many Americans are exposed to each and every day. Primarily, caffeine is found in coffee, tea, soda and chocolate. Caffeine is used to enhance power and strength and is very popular with endurance athletes. Another effect of caffeine is that during endurance activities it allows the fatty acids to be freed, thereby increasing muscle glycogen. Muscle glycogen is the fuel required for the muscles to continue contracting during physical activity. The third common side effect is an increase in the ability to fight off the effects of fatigue and drowsiness.

Caffeine does have several reported negative side effects, such as increased levels of anxiety, nervousness, irritability and insomnia. The other significant negative influence of caffeine is that it is addictive in nature. Over time the same amount of caffeine will not produce the desired effect, so more caffeine will be required by the individual. When individuals stop using caffeine in their diet it is common for them to suffer through withdrawal symptoms, and the main complaint is severe headaches.

Stimulants—The usage of stimulants may be one of the most abused drugs in all of sports. Stimulants are more widely known as amphetamines, speed, cocaine and related substances. They are used to prevent fatigue and increase alertness, speed reaction time, and the athlete's confidence.

The side effects on the body occur at the central nervous system (CNS) by increasing heart rate, blood pressure, dehydration risks, aggressiveness and anxiety. The research has not demonstrated completely that stimulants improve performance. Also, they have a significant negative effect on the athlete in activities that require a steady hand and concentration. Other negative side effects are an increase risk of strokes, cardiac irregularities (abnormal heart beats), addiction, insomnia and death.

Amino Acids—In the last 10 years, there has been a dramatic increase in the popularity of amino acids as the best nutritional supplement to increase muscle mass. The concept is that amino acids are more easily utilized and digested by the body.

Research has not supported these claims, as the body is unable to distinguish between amino acids found within food and those amino acids found in supplements. Research has also indicated that amino acids have some potential negative side effects. One possible side effect is that excessive use will cause an increased weight gain. Other negative effects are calcium loss, increase urine output, dehydration, and gout.

For most physically active Americans proper nutrition will supply the amino acids that the body requires. Americans are more inclined to believe in the quick fix, whether it be through food supplements, pills/creams that help fat dissolve or the 5 minute exercise program. To become healthier and more physically fit requires a commitment to activity and better nutrition.

Anabolic Steroids—The most commonly discussed classification of ergogenic aids is the group of drugs known as anabolic steroids. Anabolic steroids are drugs that are derivatives of the male hormone testosterone. Testosterone is required by human males to provide secondary male characteristics. It is also involved in constructive changes in the body. It increases the amino acid transfer at the cellular level which does increase musculature of the body, bone density and potential increased size of the bones.

They are injected into the body directly at the intended muscle or through the vascular system and/or taken orally. The primary reason that individuals consider involving themselves with steroids is they have a goal of increasing strength and muscle size. Many of these individuals are currently working out in a free weight setting and are not realizing their anticipated results. Other users are playing sports where size, power, strength and aggressiveness are prized commodities that could lead to a scholarship and potentially a professional contract.

The research of steroid usage is very limited due to the many potential negative side effects and the fact that it is an illegal drug. In addition it is hard to find willing participants to study over a long period of time to fully understand the implications of steroid use. The outcome of steroid use is still hotly debated, but research does indicate that steroids do increase muscle tissue growth and increase lean body mass instead of increase body fat (as with amino acids). There are also many gyms around the country where users provide non-verifiable support that increased size and muscle growth does occur. Users are primarily interested in the strength gains, increased size, and aggressiveness and are not concerned about the great number of long term negative side effects.

The side effects for males are: severe acne (usually on the back, chest, and gluteals), increase in aggressive behavior (roid rage, where the user becomes abusive/belligerent to friends, significant others, and inanimate objects), kidney damage, testicular atrophy (smaller testicles), less or ineffective sperm, enlargement of breasts, premature baldness, decreased sexual drive, premature closure of the growth plates in adolescent children, and liver damage. The other major negative effect is the early development of coronary heart disease. This outcome is relatively new and just beginning to be seriously studied. There are several reported cases of college age athletes dying from heart disease during their twenties who had no other risk factor except for steroid use. As this generation of steroid users matures, we expect to see more negative side effects develop. There also exists several additional negative side effects for females involved with steroids: masculinization, irregular menstrual cycles, a lower more masculine voice, and excessive facial and body hair.

Roid Rage should be at least discussed more thoroughly. There have been thousands of reported cases of athletes/steroid users that have literally snapped, losing control of their emotions, harming loved ones, strangers, cars, and other items. They have no control of their behavior and are very destructive. This aggressive, out of control behavior has been named "roid rage". If you are around or involved with a steroid user and they start to go off into roid rage, the best advice is to stay clear of them and remove yourself from that environment.

Another significant life threatening factor associated with steroid use is the usage of needles (works) to inject the drug into the body. Any needle usage places the individual into a high risk group for exposure to Hepatitis and HIV. As with street drugs that are injected into the body, often times the user is not concerned about sterilization of the needles. Therefore any blood that remains in the chamber/needle exposes the next person who uses the same works. If the first individual is a carrier, the second person has been exposed to either Hepatitis or the AIDS virus. Athletes that are injecting the steroids are not likely to have a constant supply of fresh, sterilized needles so reuse and sharing are likely to occur in the locker rooms and gyms. (If you are interested in this issue, check out a book called Death in the Locker Room).

These negative side effects are a serious consideration that should be thoroughly considered before anyone even thinks about using anabolic steroids.

What are some of the signs and symptoms of steroid use that the average friend, parent, coach, or teacher should be looking for? A rapid increase in muscle and weight gain in a small period of time should be viewed with suspicion. Any increase of 20-30 percent of body mass in a period of 4-8 weeks should be considered a potential positive indication of steroid use. Other signs are the severe acne, water retention (especially in the neck and facial area), a constant bad breath, and the behavioral changes previously discussed.

If you suspect drug use and the signs and symptoms tend to indicate that the potential does indeed exist, then a urinalysis would be the next step. The urinalysis should provide conclusive evidence as to usage. Then counseling may be indicated to remove the individual from the steroid cycle they became involved with.

Legally anabolic steroids are considered a controlled substance in New York state and users of the drugs without a prescription could face a Class C Felony. A conviction could lead to jail time of up to 15 years.

The following are names of the commonly available anabolic steroids. Unfortunately these are readily available on the "black" market for any one that wants to experiment and has the money.

Dianabol	Anavar	Winstrol
Danabol	Anadrol	Testred
Decca	Oranabol	

Vitamins and Minerals—The usage of vitamins and minerals has dramatically increased over the last several years. Part of this usage is related to the misconception that vitamins and minerals indeed act as an ergogenic aid. If a well balanced diet is adhered to, then the individual would not require pills to provide the essential nutrients to the body. No research has shown that increased consumption of vitamins/minerals will increase performance. Increased consumption will not lead to strength, endurance gains or for that matter any gains in the fitness/skill related areas of physical fitness.

But as discussed earlier in this chapter, Americans are constantly looking for shortcuts and view vitamins/minerals as a significant way of improving nutrition. Often the only result that the user who relies on vitamins will see is expensive urine, as most vitamin/minerals are too concentrated for the body to utilize so they are excreted.

Three other commonly used drugs that are prevalently used in society are alcohol, marijuana, and tobacco products. These drugs have been labeled "social" or recreational drugs. This is an unfortunate classification as they have harmful effects on both the physiological and psychological functions of the body.

Alcohol is not an ergogenic aid. It is a depressant that effects the central nervous system (CNS). The effects of alcohol in regards to fitness are: a decreased ability for balance activities, reaction time is slowed, small, fine motor tasks are diminished and the ability of the brain to process information is decreased. As alcohol is a legal drug that is socially accepted, it is hard to educate the millions that consume alcohol of the negative consequences. It can be safely stated that alcohol consumption before any fitness activity is foolish, as well as dangerous to the individual and those around them.

Marijuana is also not identified as an ergogenic aid, yet it affects the CNS both as a stimulant and a depressant. The effects on the body are impairment of eye/hand coordination, problems with tracking and depth perception. It is also known to change the perception of time. Another effect of marijuana is the misconception that performance is increased, when in reality the performance decreases. There is no supporting research that marijuana increases performance or that it is beneficial to any fitness activities.

The last drug that is very common in our society is tobacco. The negative effects of smoking are well documented and slowly the public is responding with no smoking areas/buildings. There is no documented evidence that smoking increases performance, although smokers refer to the relaxation effect. Smoking is on the rise in this country and especially in younger teens and adults. The ad campaigns of cigarette companies, (i.e. Joe Camel) are working and bringing new converts to tobacco.

The other area of concern with tobacco use is the increase in snuff/dipless tobacco. As young athletes watch countless hours of T.V., they inevitably see athletes using smokeless tobacco and spitting all the time. The downside of smokeless tobacco is the increased risks of cancers of the lip, mouth, esophagus and lungs, as well as the increased risk of cardiovascular disease , respiratory diseases and intestinal disease. Society must come to understand that tobacco is a potent, addictive drug, that carries serious health consequences for its users.

OTHER POTENTIAL "ERGOGENIC AIDS"

Are there ways to increase performance that do not pose serious health consequences for the individual and are socially acceptable. The answer is yes. Recently, there has been tremendous growth in the psychological approach to improving performance, whether the individual is a weekend warrior who wants to run a faster 5K race, or an elite athlete who wants to compete in the Olympics.

There are several alternatives to the previously discussed ergogenic aids. Some of them are biofeedback, relaxation training, goal setting and sport psychology.

Biofeedback is a technique that makes use of an electronic apparatus that is extremely sensitive to the physiological changes of stress in the body (increased pulse, muscle tension). If the individual can learn to lessen stress with the biofeedback machine, then he/she can use the same techniques to lessen stress during activity. This may lead to better performance when the stress is reduced to manageable levels that do not negatively affect performance.

Relaxation training is also known as progressive relaxation and involves learning a simple technique to relax the muscles. The individual learns to contract and then relax the muscle groups of the body and at the same time make use of deep breathing techniques. By relaxing the muscles, performance is often enhanced.

The use of goal setting makes the individual responsible for their actions and determine measurable outcomes. These measurable outcomes should be goals that the individual wants to achieve. By establishing these goals, it enables the individual to train and aim to achieve the goals. Specific goals are easier to obtain than "do your best" goals. The use of goal setting has been found to increase effort and lead to higher energy output toward achieving success.

FINAL THOUGHTS

Enhancing performance is a normal thought process for any weekend warrior. The hope is that more people will use healthier aids in the future. The focus of this chapter was to introduce ergogenic aids and discuss both negative and positive side effects. The exact benefit of ergogenic aids is often not fully understood by the user, but they are willing to try for the quick and easy results. It is important to understand that if an individual is looking for better performance, the newer psychological approach has shown great potential and promise. If a person is looking to improve their fitness level, they should make a commitment to follow the FIT concept, improve their nutrition, allow for play each and every day and reduce stress in their lives.

WORKSHEET 14-A

Chapter Fourteen—Ergogenic Aids

Matching: Put the letter of the definition next to the word/phrase.

Words/Phrases

1. Ergogenic Aid   1. _____
2. Increase in muscle size   2. _____
3. Increase in muscle strength   3. _____
4. Increase in competitive attitude   4. _____
5. Lower pain perception   5. _____
6. "Roid rage"   6. _____
7. Addiction   7. _____
8. Severe acne   8. _____
9. Testicular atrophy   9. _____
10. Impotence and sterility   10. _____
11. Interruption of menstrual cycle   11. _____
12. Facial and torso hair growth   12. _____
13. Premature baldness   13. _____
14. Heart disease   14. _____
15. Cancer   15. _____
16. Anabolic Steroid   16. _____
17. Caffeine   17. _____
18. Nicotine   18. _____
19. Ethol alcohol   19. _____
20. Biofeedback   20. _____
21. Guided imagery   21. _____
22. Goal setting   22. _____
23. Vitamin   23. _____
24. Mineral   24. _____
25. Amino acid   25. _____

Definitions

A. Nutritional supplement with no proven ergogenic benefit.
B. Nutritional supplement with no proven ergogenic benefit.
C. Psychological training having the person visualize a successful task completion.
D. CNS depressant with no proven ergogenic benefit.
E. CNS stimulant with no proven ergogenic benefit.
F. Reported life threatening possible adverse effect of steroid abuse.
G. Reported side effect for both male and female steroid abuse.
H. Reported side effect for female steroid abuse.
I. Reported side effect for male steroid abuse.
J. Reported side effect for male and female steroid abuse.
K. Perceived benefit of steroid use.

L. Perceived benefit of steroid use.

M. Substances taken as a supplement that purport to improve physical performance.

N. Nutritional supplement with no proven ergogenic benefit.

O. Psychological training using specific objectives/targets.

P. Psychological training to recognize the reactions of the body.

Q. CNS stimulant with no proven ergogenic benefit.

R. Testosterone derivative hormone with tissue building function.

S. Reported life threatening possible adverse effect of steroid abuse.

T. Reported side effect of male and female steroid abuse.

U. Reported side effect of male steroid abuse.

V. Reported side effect of male and female steroid abuse.

W. Reported psychological side effect for male and female steroid abuse.

X. Perceived benefit of steroid use.

Y. Perceived benefit of steroid use.

CHAPTER FIFTEEN
Back Care

Outside of the common cold, back problems are the most common complaint of Americans. It is estimated that at some time or another, 80% of the adult population will experience some degree of back problems, with the 20-45 age group the most frequently afflicted.

Back problems are also the most expensive in terms of a loss of productivity and compensation case settlements to business and industry.

The obvious question of course is WHY? The reasons are many and will be addressed at length later in the chapter. But first in order to better understand the reasons and be able to affect positive change, a basic explanation of the structure and function of the human spinal column will be presented.

STRUCTURE

The human back is a series of individual bones stacked one atop the other (see Figure 15-1). These bones are called vertebrae and are separated by cartilage pads called discs, which prevent the two hard boney surfaces from contacting each other. There are a total of 33 individual vertebrae, with 24 being movable and 9 fused (see Figure 15-2).

The vertebral size is specific to the site. The vertebrae are smallest in the neck and get progressively larger as they approach the lumbar area just above the pelvic girdle. It appears that the more weight required to be supported determines the size of the vertebrae in that area.

Cervical   —   7

Thoracic   —   12

Lumbar   —   5

Sacral   —   5*

Coccygeal   —   4*

TOTAL   —   33
*Fused

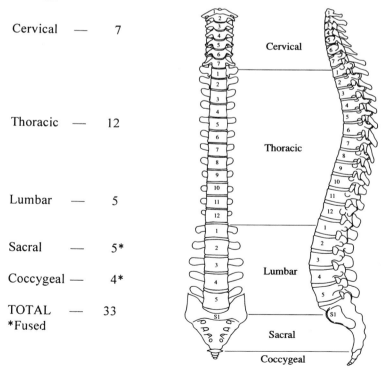

Figure 15-1 Vertebral Column

FUNCTION

The function of the spinal column is to protect the spinal cord, which is the extension of the brain that runs through the length of the stacked vertebrae. The spinal cord contains all of the nerves that controls all of the functions of the body.

MOVEMENT

Each individual vertebrae moves a little bit. But in concert with the rest of the spinal column, they can create a wide range of motion. Of similar importance is the fact that each individual vertebral joint is involved in almost all movements. Therefore, an injury to one vertebral joint is not going to be limited to that joint only. It will have an adverse impact on all movements.

The normal movements of the spine are flexion (bending) extension (straightening), hyperextension (arching back), lateral flexion (side bending) and rotation (turning).

If these actions are performed mechanically correct, while in balance and without an overload, they are all relatively safe. However if done incorrectly, or while out of balance or with an inappropriate overload, they can be very dangerous.

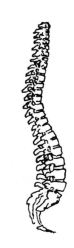

Figure 15-2 Vertebrae

DISC MOVEMENT

The shock absorbing discs encounter different mechanical stresses depending on the movement. In simple bending at the waist (Flexion), the front of the disc is compressed while the back is pulled apart under tension (See Figure 15-3). The reverse would be true in extension or straightening at the waist. Rotation or twisitng creates a shearing force within the joint (See Figure 15-4). These simple movements create vulnerable positions at certain times within the joint. It wouldn't be a recommended practice to bend over and twist the torso at the same time. This would combine all three forces simultaneously within a joint.

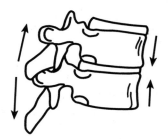

Figure 15-3 Compression Tension

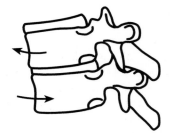

Figure 15-4 Shearing

COMMON CAUSES OF BACK PROBLEMS

Aging

The aging process reduces the elasticity of the connective tissues of the back. The loss of this elasticity in the tendons, muscles and ligaments reduces the flexibility and range of motion of each joint. Therefore stresses in the form of forced range of motion become a problem for the aging back. When younger, these movements would present no problem, but because of a loss of flexibility through aging, these same movements can be an injury mechanism.

The aging process also reduces bone density rendering the vertebrae more vulnerable to stress fractures. This is called osteoporosis and results in the bones becoming more brittle because they become more hollow. Osteoporosis is a very common problem for middle to senior age females. Again actions or motions performed by the senior citizen can become injury mechanisms, even though they can be safely performed by younger people. The stresses of the action are not as easily dissipated in an aging back.

Another effect of aging is that the discs between the bones become less resilient through a loss of water absorption capability. This has the net effect of reducing the shock absorbing function of the cartilage pads. This reduces height, changes posture angles and offers less protection to the bony surfaces of the vertebrae.

Posture

The back has a series of normal curves (See Figure 15-5) that enable it to function mechanically safe and effective. The back of the neck and low back curve in from the posterior, and the shoulder blades and buttocks curve out. Any change in these normal curves puts undo mechanical stress on the connective tissues of the vertebral column. This can result in damage to these tissue as they are now called upon to function is a manner in which they were not designed.

By maintaining proper posture the spine is balanced, and the mechanical stresses are reduced. Therefore it is recommended that postural awareness be an essential component of any physical work or activity/exercise program. It is undesirable to ask the connective tissue to compensate for poor posture at rest. And it is simply dangerous to ask the tissue to do the same under the stresses of physical labor or activity/exercise.

To ensure proper posture, a very good check list to follow is to ask oneself these questions:

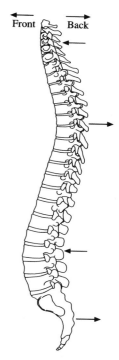

Front   Back

> *"Is my head over my shoulders?"*
> *"Are my shoulders over my hips?"*
> *"Are my hips over my feet?"*

If they are, the vertebral column is as close as it can be expected to its' normal curve alignment. This makes the posture or action as safe as can be expected. If not, abnormal mechanical stresses have been created placing the spine in a less than ideal functional position.

Figure 15-5 Spinal Curves

Flexibility

A loss of flexibility in certain musculature can cause low back problems. The hamstring group which is behind the thigh and runs from the pelvic girdle to the lower leg is of particular concern. If this muscle group is too tight, it causes the pelvic girdle to be tilted backward flattening out the curve in the lower back.

This creates mechanical stress in the lumbar/sacral area and in particular the first movable joint in L5/S1.

Muscular Strength

A loss of muscular strength particularly in the abdominal area can also cause abnormal mechanical stress. This time the stress is caused by hyperextension or an exaggerated low back curve. This creates undo tension in the front of the disc and compression in the back. The imbalance puts a great deal of stress on the connective tissue in the low back in order to compensate for the misalignment. The abdominal muscles have a major supportive function for the spine. Deconditioning or distension of the musculature ("Beer Belly" or pregnancy) is often associated with low back pain.

The same holds true for the hip flexors which are responsible for stabilizing the pelvic girdle. Weakness in these muscles will also contribute to the exaggerated forward pelvic tilt. Weakness in the extensors of the back and the retractors of the shoulder create the "stooped over" appearance that is actually a form of spinal imbalance. The stress created by this muscle weakness also places undo strain on the low back connective tissue as it attempts to compensate for the poor posture created by the muscle weakness.

Overfat/Obesity

Non productive tissue creates excessive stress on the back in two ways—support and movement. More weight simply creates an overload on the structures of the back. This excess weight is a stress in itself.

This overload problem is compounded by the fact that the excessive weight creates an imbalance in the spine which must be compensated for by other connective tissue, placing them under stress.

This combination adversely effects the stability of the spine and increases the risk of injury.

Poor Mechanics

Often times back problems are caused by the person simply performing work or activities while in the wrong position. The basic rule is that the back is not a lever, the arms and legs are. Humans are designed to do work with the levers not the back. The back is the stabilizer or the point around which action should occur. The back should not be used to perform the work.

However this rule is not followed in many cases, and the result is undo stress being placed on the vertebral column. This can occur in a one time acute action or in a series of low intensity repetitive actions. In either case, the back was made to do the work that the arms and legs should be doing.

A good example of this is the simple lift task. Simple lifting tasks should be done with the legs not the back. Whether it is a one time high intensity action, such as furniture moving, or repetitive actions, such as a grocery clerk transferring grocery bags from the check out counter to shopping cart, each can be an injury mechanism to the back if done incorrectly.

Another common mechanical cause of back problems is the combining of actions while under stress. Flexing the vertebral column while rotating creates compression, tension and shear forces simultaneously. Therefore doing high intensity or overload work in this position would make the discs vulnerable.

The example would be to bend over at the waist and then twist one way or the other to pick up a heavy object.

RECOMMENDED BACK EXERCISES—PREVENTATIVE MAINTENANCE

For each of the following exercises refer to the numbered photographs on the facing page.

1. Trunk Rotation
2. Low Back Rotation
3. Overcorrect
4. Pelvic Tilt
5. Knee to Chest
6. Hamstring Stretch
7. Crunch
8. Prone upper Back Extension
9. Prone Arm & Leg Extension
10. All Fours Arm & Leg Extension

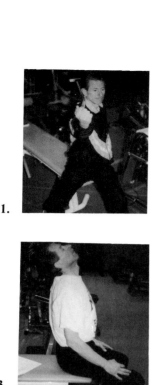

1.

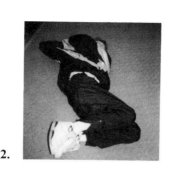

2.

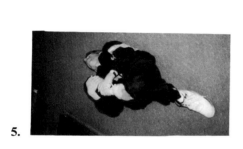

3.

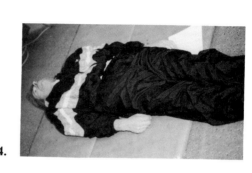

4.

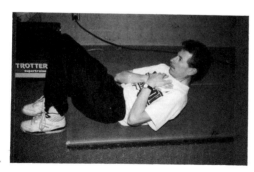

5.

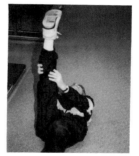

6.

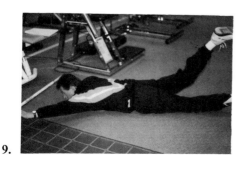

7.

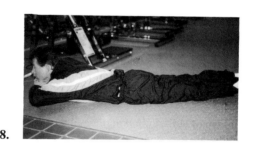

8.

9.

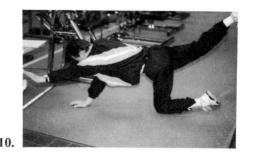

10.

Recommendations for Back Care

Standing

If forced to stand stationary, place one foot in front of the other and on a slightly elevated surface. (Stool, step, etc.) Use work surfaces at an appropriate height. Do not bend over to work while standing.

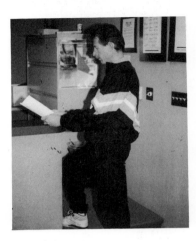 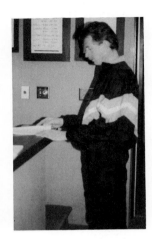

Sitting

Sit straight, facing forward. Keep the feet flat and the back against the backrest of the chair. Keep the head over shoulders and stay close to the work surface to avoid reaching.

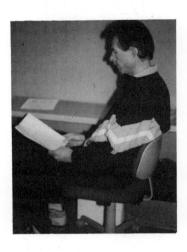 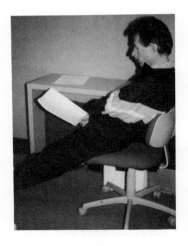

Bending

Only bend forward from the waist while slightly bending the knees. Don't stoop or bend over from the waist only.

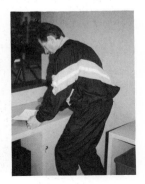 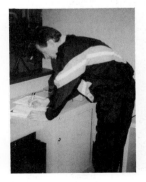

Reaching

Only reach forward. Don't reach and twist. Don't reach and attempt to lift. Don't reach and attempt to catch something. Don't reach and attempt to apply force.

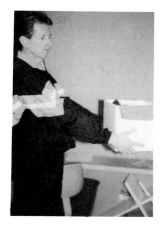 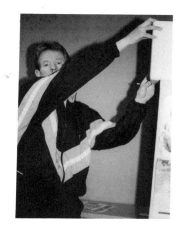

Carrying

Don't carry things away from the body. Carry things as close to the body as possible. Don't overload one side of the body while carrying.

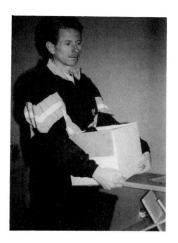 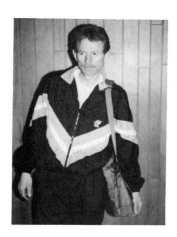

Lifting

Lift things off the floor with a bent knee, not bent over at the waist. Keep back straight and raise object with the legs. If turning or twisting is required, turn the body by turning the feet not by turning the trunk.

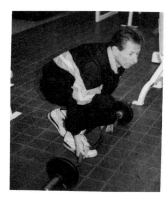 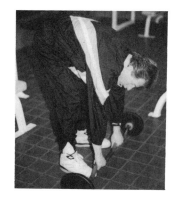

Push Pull

Only push or pull objects using the arms and legs. Don't use the bending/straightening action at the waist as a force application method.

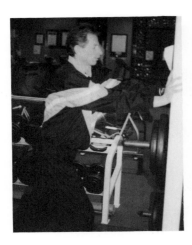 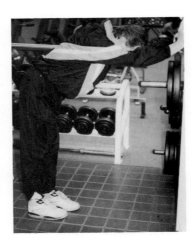

Sleeping/Lying

Don't sleep lying on the back with feet level with the body. If this position is desirable, elevate the legs to a semi hip and knee flex position by placing something underneath the knees which will elevate them 8-10 inches.

Don't sleep lying face down.

Don't sleep lying on your side in a straight leg position. Bend the knees and the hips and keep the arms down below the head.

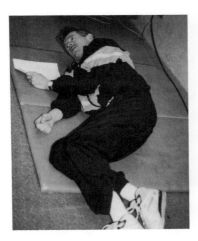 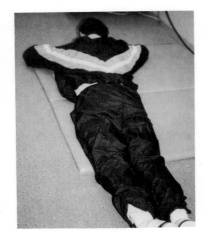

WORKSHEET 15-A

Chapter Fifteen—Back Care

MONROE COMMUNITY COLLEGE BACK EVALUATION SURVEY

INSTRUCTIONS: Select the word that best represents you in response to the statement. Write the points assigned to that selection in the points column. Total the column at the end of the survey. Consult the back risk evaluation chart listed at the end of the survey to get the interpretation of your score.

KEY: A—Always,   RG—Regularly,   S—Sometimes,   RR—Rarely,   N—Never.

STATEMENT	POINTS
1. I engage in a formal exercise routine. A—1, RG—2, S—3, RR—4, N—5	1._____
2. I am in the acceptable range for body fat %. A—1, RG—2, S—3, RR—4, N—5	2._____
3. I stand in a stationary position for long periods of time. A—5, RG—4, S—3, RR—2, N—1	3._____
4. I sit in a stationary position for long periods of time. A—5, RG—4, S—3, RR—2, N—1	4._____
5. I sit with both feet flat on the floor. A—1, RG—2, S—3, RR—4, N—5	5._____
6. I sit with my back up against the backrest. A—1, RG—2, S—3, RR—4, N—5	6._____
7. When I sit, I reach, stretch and twist to do my work. A—5, RG—4, S—3, RR—2, N—1	7._____
8. When I drive, I move the seat back as far as possible. A—5, RG—4, S—3, RR—2, N—1	8._____
9. When I carry something, I carry it as close to the body as possible. A—1, RG—2, S—3, RR—4, N—5	9._____
10. When I carry something, I balance it on both sides on my body. A—1, RG—2, S—3, RR—4, N—5	10._____
11. When I lift something, I use my legs. A—1, RG—2, S—3, RR—4, N—5	11._____
12. When I lift something, I twist and turn while doing it. A—5, RG—4, S—3, RR—2, N—1	12._____
13. My job requires me to lift heavy objects. A—5, RG—4, S—3, RR—2, N—1	13._____
14. My job requires me to lift lighter objects continually. A—5, RG—4, S—3, RR—2, N—1	14._____

15. I sleep on my stomach.
A—5, RG—4, S—3, RR—2, N—1

15._____

16. I sleep on my back.
A—5, RG—4, S—3, RR—2, N—1

16._____

17. I sleep on a very soft mattress/surface.
A—5, RG—4, S—3, RR—2, N—1

17._____

18. My job requires me to do a lot of pushing.
A—5, RG—4, S—3, RR—2, N—1

18._____

19. My job requires me to do a lot of pulling.
A—5, RG—4, S—3, RR—2, N—1

19._____

20. I am conscious of my posture.
A—1, RG—2, S—3, RR—4, N—5

20._____

21. I eat a balanced mixed diet.
A—1, RG—2, S—3, RR—4, N—5

21._____

22. My age is
1—20-29, 2—30-39, 3—40-49, 4—50-59, 5—60-69

22._____

BACK RISK EVALUATION CHART

POINT TOTAL	RISK
101 — 110	HIGH
76 — 100	ABOVE AVERAGE
36 — 75	AVERAGE
11 — 35	BELOW AVERAGE
0 — 10	LOW

CHAPTER SIXTEEN
Stress and Stress Management

In today's world, we are all influenced by overwhelming expectations and responsibilities that at times become too much. One of the least understood and least recognized health risks that face all of us is stress. I always ask the students in my classrooms, how many of you are under stress? The response is always small, yet many of them are under significant amounts of stress and don't even realize it. The student's stress comes from many areas such as attending college, working, being involved with a significant other, being a parent, living with their parents, and often a combination of several of the preceding. The students deal with these situations and often are unsure as how they influence the amount of stress in their lives. Even if they were able to identify the stressors in their lives, a sense of hopelessness stills exist. This feeling comes from the fact that we have lost control and are unsure of how to defuse the stress in our lives. It is unfortunate that in today's society STRESS is commonplace and little is done to further understand it's impact. The focus of this chapter will be to introduce stress, understand the effects on the body, and begin the concept of replacing stress with healthful alternatives.

As we discuss stress, we should have a definition to frame the concepts presented within this chapter. Stress is a bodily response to any stimulus (usually negative) that elicits a change/effect within our body. Often times these responses are increased blood pressure, nervousness, agitation, anger, sweating palms, racing heart, headaches and others. The changes that occur within our bodies are often varied depending on the stressor and our frame of mind at that particular time. Examples of stressful situations can range from the surprise pop quiz the professor just announced; to almost being in a car accident; to finding out that a friend just died; to your wedding day. Any of these situations may have produced a reaction within your body. Whether the example was perceived as either negative or positive, a response was produced within your body.

Before preceding, answer the following questions about yourself. These questions and your responses will help formulate a groundwork to build upon. Answer Yes or No.

1. Are you often angry, frustrated, tense and unsure of how to handle it?
2. Have you ever lost it (yelled, gotten physical) with a significant other?
3. Do you get headaches, upset stomachs, when you are overwhelmed or stressed out?
4. Do you feel as if you have lost control of your life?
5. At night, when you sleep would you say that it is a restful sleep?
6. Do you get at least 7-8 hours a sleep a night?
7. Do you work more than 1 job, or are you a parent going to school?
8. Do you find time on a regular basis for play, recreational activities, and or exercise?

If you answered yes, to questions 1,2,3,4,7 and no to 5, 6, and 8, then there is some indication that stress does exist within your world. Now that you are aware of stress in your lives, you must come to a better understanding of what that means.

As we discuss stress, it will be important to understand where stress comes from. Humans are bombarded every day of their lives with stressors. These stressors can be placed within three categories: environmental, physiological and psycho-social.

1. **Environmental**—These stressors come from the places we live, work, go to school and play. Examples are overcrowding, heat, noise, weather, cold, anything that affects our living environment. Another example of an environmental stressors would be living in Rochester. During the winter, we start with excitement over the first snow and remark how pretty it makes the world. By the end of January, we are complaining about the cold, snow and hope that

spring is coming soon. In March, we are irritable over the cold, the mounds of snow and hope that Spring and sunshine will follow soon. There are several studies that investigate how the lack of sunshine affects our well being and health. Think about how much better we all feel when the sun is out, especially in the middle of the winter.

2. **Physiological**—These stressors are illnesses and injuries that affect our bodies. Obviously, there exists many types of injuries and illnesses that affect all of us. Usually, this category consists of long term injuries or diseases that are of sudden onset and of serious consequence. It is also important to understand that each and every one of us reacts differently to all stressors.

3. **Psycho-social**—Probably the category that most of us are aware of. Examples of psycho-social stressors are: losing your job, divorce, death of a close friend/family member, moving to a new town, going to college, and any other major change in our life events. These changes are significant to the person and are seen as having a dramatic impact on their lives. Again, what someone may see as a tremendous opportunity, someone else may feel as if the end of the world is coming.

We must understand that every day we are being exposed to a variety of stressors and often we are unaware of the significant influences they provide. To remain in control of our lives, we must acknowledge that stress exists, be aware of its effects and learn to control stress before it controls us.

Stress has been with us since prehistoric man, and we still have the same mechanism for dealing with stress as early man. That system is the Fight or Flight response which is the body's defensive response to stress. For prehistoric man, stress came from providing food for the family/clan, protecting yourself from wild animals, and others. As civilization has progressed, the stressors that are bombarding us every day have increased and yet have not really changed all that much. We still are concerned with feeding our family, protecting ourselves, working, living, and yet we have not learned to manage stress any better.

STRESS MANAGEMENT

The biggest factor in dealing with stress is identifying that it has a role in your life. Some stress is important and beneficial to us. It provides us with the drive to solve problems, increase productivity and keeps us active and involved. There are three different levels of stress that should be addressed: eustress, rust-out, and burn-out. Eustress is what is normal for each of us. The problem is, what is meant by normal. Every individual perceives and reacts differently to stress. What is normal to you may push another individual over the edge. Eustress is the amount of stress in your life that is not having a negative effect or causing problems for you.

Rust-out is a term that is not often used within our high paced, cram it all in society of the 90's. The concept of rust-out is for the individual that is not experiencing stress within their lives. Without stress, the fight or flight system is not used often and thereby does not function well when it is truly needed (Like a rusty old water faucet that has not been used often, the spigot over time starts to rust from disuse). Rust-out is not a major factor when discussing stress in America.

Burn-out is the last classification of stress. This term has its roots in the paramedical field of emergency care. The pioneer paramedics were required to work long shifts, see incredible injuries that were often life threatening, and never know whether their work was beneficial. It was fairly common for the paramedics to experience work/social problems related to their jobs, i.e. a high turnover on the job, divorce rate was higher and an increase in the suicide rate when compared to other groups. For paramedics having these similar problems, burn-out was the name given. In today's society, the burn-out label is not given just to paramedics. It is used to describe the feelings of loss, and out of control behavior that is exhibited by countless thousands of professionals, students, and every day people.

Burn-out has been replaced today by the term distress. Distress indicates long or extended periods of unvaried stress and frustration levels that become negative/harmful.

HOW DO YOU HANDLE STRESS?????? On the lines that follow, develop two lists. The list on the left hand side is for negative ways that you can think of to handle stress. On the right hand column, identify any positive ways to handle stress.

Negative	**Positive**
_____	_____
_____	_____
_____	_____

_____   _____

_____   _____

_____   _____

_____   _____

_____   _____

The following are some of the behaviors that previous students have developed for dealing with stress and comments about each. Do you find yourself in any of these? If you did, you are probably not managing your stress very well.

   a. All abusive behavior (spousal, child, physical, verbal)—where the individual attempts to feel better by lowering those around them.
   b. Drinking/drug use—seen as an escape from the pressures of stress, yet when you come down from the drug or get over the hangover, the problem still exists and you may have compounded it while under the influence of the drug.
   c. Shopping—at the time you may enjoy it and will make you feel better, but what happens when you spent food money, or charged it with no reasonable expectations of being able to pay the bill at any time soon.
   d. Driving a car—have you ever been driving a car and some other driver cuts you off, what is your initial reaction, do you flip them off, do you race up and tailgate, or do you pass them and cut them off. A car is not a good place to be angry and trying to get even. We tend to drive fast, disobey the law and drive crazy.
   e. Suicide—obviously the strongest reaction to stress and to the feelings of being out of control. Suicide is usually an unplanned immediate response to the situation and often cannot be reversed. It would be hard to imagine many situations where suicide would appear to be a realistic manner of solving the problem. Unfortunately, those individuals who commit suicide view it as solving or removing themselves from the pain, frustration, hurt of their lives.
   f. Sex—If sex is used to deal with stress, unfortunately the outcome can often cause more stress. Questions are raised about selfishness and safety.
   g. Sleep—can be viewed as an escape mechanism so therefore is placed on the negative side. When sleep becomes the primary outcome of our lives, it is being used to avoid our problems in the hope that they will disappear.
   h. Anger—have you ever witnessed a parent in a restaurant lose control when his/her child spilled a drink. The outcomes are obvious. The parent has reached his/her boiling point, blood pressure is increased, face is red and tense, and the child is quivering and in tears.

On the other hand, the following is a list of positive responses. Do you find yourself in any of these? If you do, it means that you are managing stress very well.

   a. Exercise/play—is the most beneficial manner of dealing with the stress in our lives. With exercise we can remove the negative energy that is given off by stress and use it for the benefit of our bodies. Exercise allows us the perfect opportunity to displace our frustration and remove the anger that is within.
   b. Talking to someone—by talking to a friend, minister, loved one, teacher, you are able to get it off your chest and get another perspective on the situation. It helps to see it from someone else's side.
   c. Hobbies—this provides some quiet time away from the rat race and allows you a chance to calm down and defuse yourself. Hobbies can range from woodworking, gardening, sewing, baking, models, knitting, to reading and writing poetry.
   d. Watching a sunrise/sunset, enjoying the outdoors—think back to the last time you watched a sunset. Remember the incredible colors and beauty. Close your eyes and paint the picture in your mind. Do you feel the inner calm and serenity. Many of us have become so busy with work and keeping up with the Jones that we have forgot how to enjoy the simpler things around us.
   e. Music—put your favorite CD/tape on. Each of us has our favorite music that refreshes us and makes us feel better. For some it may be new age, jazz, country, rock & roll, rap. If it makes you feel better then utilize it.

f. Take a vacation—many of us look forward to a vacation based on the fact that we are leaving work and getting away. Although sometimes a vacation may increase our stress level, with a few simple changes we can lower our stress levels. Don't rush out of town Friday afternoon. Leave Saturday, after you have caught up with all loose tasks. Come home a day early so you can go through the mail, go grocery shopping and unwind from your vacation. Plan short vacations, i.e. long weekends throughout the year instead of 2 vacations (summer and winter).

g. Crying—why would this be placed here (the men are saying). It isn't a sign of weakness, and for many it is a good way to release the energy and emotions that have built up.

h. Massage, Yoga, T.M., and other relaxation techniques—each of these activities allows the individual to become more in tune with his/her body. These activities allow for an inner calm and peace to come about, as well as increasing mental alertness.

As you review your list of ways of dealing with stress, do you most often choose from the positive or negative side? If you constantly choose from the negative side, then you may unknowingly be increasing your stress level. Review your lists and start to examine if other possibilities exist for your individual stress management.

In conclusion, please consider the following list of recommendations for stress management.

a. Never keep it inside, find an outlet for the frustration and anger. Work it off, exercise but find an outlet so as not to keep it bottled up.

b. Escape for a while, find a place that provides a time for reflection, quiet time where you won't be disturbed.

c. Involve a friend, talk to them about what is bothering you. Let others help you, it is not you against the rest of the world.

d. Become better at time management. Know your capabilities and work within them. If you can't do something, then don't volunteer. It only increases the stress you place on yourself. You are not superman/woman, so don't try to be.

e. Do unto others as you would have them do unto you. The ability to help others not only provides a good feeling for you, but it also allows you the opportunity to forget about your problems for a period of time. Additionally, it reminds us that others may have worse problems then our own or that our problems seem somewhat petty.

f. Give praise to others and to yourself. If you did a good job, whether at work, school or home and no one notices, go ahead and say good job. Don't rely on others to always praise you, learn to give and believe in your own praise.

g. Reduce criticism of others. Be more tolerant of individual differences.

h. Never forget to tell those you care about, that you do love or care for them. Life is too short to leave those around us guessing about our feelings and our intentions. Show feelings and emotions.

i. Remember to play each and every day of our lives. Those that are active and full of energy have embraced each day as a treasure and make the most of it. Play often, enjoy exercise as a vital ingredient to a happy, fulfilled life.

j. Smile more and frown less. Provide a positive, upbeat, warm, caring, environment for friends and colleagues. It has to start with someone, so make that someone YOU.

k. Live life in the present and clear your mind of past events, especially unpleasant memories. Enjoy the present moment before it to becomes a memory.

l. Remember to laugh. Laughter is a very good stress reliever and provides an outlet for you.

m. Develop moderate expectations of yourself and those around you. If the expectations are too high, it only increases the stress in your life. In addition, develop the ability to go with the flow. This simply means to be flexible and view all challenges as exciting, new ways to learn and grow.

WORKSHEET 16-A

Chapter Sixteen—How Vulnerable are You to Stress

As discussed within this chapter, a wide variety of stressors are bombarding us all the time. These stressors are identified as either environmental, physiological, or psycho-social. This lab will identify certain perceived stressful situations and assign a point value for each. By answering truthfully we will attempt to assess your overall vulnerability to stress. The scoring system is as follows.

1= always (yes)   2 = almost always   3 = most of the time   4 = some of the time   5 = never (no)

Situation   **Score**

I get the appropriate amount of sleep my body needs to function.   _____

I exercise to perspiration at least twice a week   _____

I do not smoke, or I smoke less than half a pack a day   _____

I regularly attend club or social activities   _____

I have at least 1 friend to confide in regarding personal matters.   _____

I am able to vent my feelings when angry or worried.   _____

I am able to organize my time effectively.   _____

I drink fewer than 3 cups of coffee (or tea, cola drinks) a day.   _____

I take quiet time for myself during the day.   _____

I do not procrastinate, I get things done right away.   _____

Before a test I get to bed at the same time I normally would.   _____

I live at home (with my family or spouse) while attending school.   _____

I try not to let other people's problems become my own.   _____

If sexually active, I practice safe sex.   _____

The people closest to me are supportive of my goals.   _____

I have money to meet recreational activities.   _____

I am attending college by choice.   _____

I rarely compare myself with my friends.   _____

I do not hold a job and go to school full time.   _____

My G.P.A. is set only for personal satisfaction.   _____

I do not plan on going on to higher levels of education.   _____

                                                              Total: _____

SCORING: Your Total Point Value _____ -20 = _____ Final Score

Interpretation: 30-49 points =   Vulnerable to stress

                       50-75 points =   Seriously vulnerable to stress

                       76-105 points =   Extremely vulnerable to stress

WORKSHEET 16-B
WORKPLACE BEHAVIOR SELF EVALUATION

1—NEVER;   2—RARELY;   3—SOMETIMES; 4—OFTEN;   5—ALWAYS.

1. I know exactly what my job description is.   1. _____

2. I find out the formal line and staff order.   2. _____

3. I follow the line and staff order.   3. _____

4. If I don't understand/know something I need to know to do my job, I ask questions.   4. _____

5. I fulfill my job description on a daily basis.   5. _____

6. I demonstrate a reasonable level of interest in my job.   6. _____

7. I demonstrate a reasonable level of enthusiasm for my job.   7. _____

8. I am willing to occasionally do more than I am required to do.   8. _____

9. I am on time.   9. _____

10. I am prepared.   10. _____

11. I limit my tendency to complain.   11. _____

12. I know when to complain and when not to.   12. _____

13. I try to solve minor complaints myself.   13. _____

14. I can control my emotions.   14. _____

15. I try to learn from my mistakes so as not to repeat them.   15. _____

16. I try to accept constructive criticism.   16. _____

17. I am very careful about saying negative things about colleagues and superiors.   17. _____

18. If I complain, I make it about the process not the person.   18. _____

19. I acknowledge assistance with a form of a thank you.   19. _____

20. I only make commitments I intend to keep.   20. _____

21. My word is good.   21. _____

22. I praise/recognize people when they earn it.   22. _____

23. I share ideas/materials/facilities willingly.   23. _____

24. When slighted/offended, I control the urge to seek revenge.   24. _____

25. I don't let other people trigger me.   25. _____

26. I don't let other people intimidate me.   26. _____

27. I avoid minor confrontations.   27. _____

28. I address major confrontations.   28. _____

29. I can laugh at myself.   29. _____

30. I recognize time wasters.   30. _____

31. I recognize time savers.   31. _____

32. I believe in personal development.   32. _____

33. I am not resentful/envious of others successes.   33. _____

34. I don't try to do things that I know I am not capable of doing.   34. _____

35. I don't claim others work as my own.   35. _____

36. I respect the opinion of others.   36. _____

37. I know the difference between personal and professional.   37. _____

38. I regularly evaluate my position/performance.   38. _____

39. I critically evaluate my work.   39. _____

40. I have a life outside of work.   40. _____

41. I cooperate with my colleagues.   41. _____

42. I am considerate of my colleagues.   42. _____

43. I practice personal development.   43. _____

44. I embrace change.   44. _____

45. I am willing to listen to dissenting opinions.   45. _____

46. I willingly help my colleagues.   46. _____

47. I can readily adapt to a changing environment.   47. _____

48. I am a good listener.   48. _____

49. I problem solve.   49. _____

50. Honesty is the best policy.   50. _____

EVALUATION

    0—42   Problem waiting to happen.

  43—85   Low producer/contributor, frequent problems.

  86—169   Average employee. Problems and contributions are few.

170—210   Contributor/producer with rare problems.

211—250   Positive, top producer/contributor, innovative and current.

CHAPTER SEVENTEEN
Hypokinetic Disease

The human body was designed to be physically active. Early man had to depend upon his physical skills for food, clothing and shelter. These conditions continued for many years. Today we have developed labor saving devices for nearly every task. Most of our occupations require little or no physical effort. In addition our eating habits have changed drastically with processed foods and fast food restaurants.

Despite the fact that our current lifestyles require little or no physical activity, our bodies still require movement to maintain health and fitness. Hypokinetic diseases have replaced infectious diseases as the major causes of death. Hypokinetic diseases are those diseases that are related to, or caused by, a lack of regular physical activity. Heart disease, obesity, high blood pressure, low-back pain, cancer and osteoporosis are examples of these diseases and conditions.

CARDIOVASCULAR DISEASE

Cardiovascular disease are the most prevalent degenerative disease in the United States. These are diseases which affect the heart and circulatory system. Cardiovascular disease results in as many deaths, each year, as all other causes of death combined.

In 1985 disease of the heart and blood vessels had a cost in excess of 80 billion dollars. 132 million workdays are lost annually because of this disease.

Approximately 50 percent of those who suffer some form of coronary heart disease will suffer a heart attack. This heart attack will be the first symptom of the disease. Forty percent of those who suffer heart attack die within the first 24 hours. Forty percent of those who die are in the age group thirty to sixty-five.

In most cardiovascular diseases we do not know the specific cause. There is no absolute method to prevent cardiovascular disease. There are, however, methods to reduce one's risk of suffering from these diseases.

CORONARY ARTERY DISEASE

Coronary Artery Disease is the most common form of cardiovascular disease. It is characterized by a reduction in the opening of coronary arteries. These are the blood vessels which supply the heart muscle with it's blood and oxygen supply.

Atherosclerosis is a progressive condition which contributes to coronary artery disease. Lesions develop in the walls of the coronary arteries. They are composed of cholesterol, lipids, blood cells and calcium. This plaque begins to accumulate in early childhood and continues throughout one's lifetime. Ultimately it reduces or cuts off blood flow to the heart.

Normal Artery   Inner Wall Deposits   Hardened Deposits

Figure 17-1

Angina Pectoris means chest pain. It is caused by the inability of the coronary arteries to supply the heart muscle with an adequate oxygen supply. It most often occurs during activity and subsides when activity stops.

Myocardial Infarction means the death of heart muscle tissue. Commonly called a heart attack, it occurs when an obstruction or spasm disrupts or terminates the flow of blood to a portion of the heart. Heart muscle cells deprived of oxygen die. The location of the obstruction or spasm determines the amount of muscle tissue damage. This is an irreversible injury since the scar tissue which forms can no longer contribute to the pumping of blood.

Risk Factors

In most cases the cause of cardiovascular disease is unknown. There are conditions which increase a person's risk of suffering a cardiovascular event. These are called risk factors.

Unchangeable Risk Factors are those risk factors that people are born with. They can not be changed by lifestyle changes. They include increased age, male sex and family history and race.

Changeable Risk Factors are those that can be changed by changes in a person's lifestyle. They include elevated blood cholesterol, hypertension, cigarette smoking, a lack of physical activity, obesity, glucose intolerance and stress.

Chapter 11 has additional information about risk factor reduction.

Signs of Heart Attack

1. Uncomfortable fullness, squeezing or pressure in and around the chest, or pain in the center of the chest lasting for several minutes.
2. Pain that spreads to the shoulder, arms or neck.
3. The above accompanied by one or more of following, dizziness, fainting, sweating, nausea or shortness of breath.

STROKE

The majority of strokes are similar to coronary artery disease except that they occur in the brain instead of the heart. There are five basic causes of strokes.

A **thrombus** is a clot that forms to prevent blood flow through an artery to brain tissue.

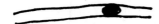

Figure 17-2 Thrombus

An **embolism** is a clot that has formed elsewhere in the body. It travels through the arterial system and becomes lodged in the smaller cerebral blood vessels.

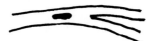

Figure 17-3 Embolism

Cerebral hemorrhage occurs when a cerebral blood vessel bursts. This most often occurs due to an aneurysm (a weak spot in the artery that expands like a balloon and bursts under pressure.

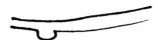

Figure 17-4 Aneurysm

A **compression** is usually an outside force (tumor) which collapses the artery wall preventing the flow of blood.

Figure 17-5 Compression

A **spasm** is the constriction of the artery when the smooth muscle tissue in the artery wall contracts, thus narrowing the artery and reducing blood flow.

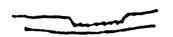

Figure 17-6 Spasm

Brain tissue deprived of oxygen dies. The body functions controlled by the affected portion of the brain become nonfunctional. These include paralysis, speech impediments and loss of memory.

Signs and Symptoms of a Stroke
1. Temporary loss of speech, difficulty in speaking of understanding speech.
2. Unexplained dizziness, unsteadiness or sudden falls.
3. Temporary dimness or loss of vision.
4. Sudden, temporary weakness or numbness of the face, arm and leg on one side of the body.

HYPERTENSION

Blood pressure is the force exerted against the walls of the arteries and the resistance to blood flow by the arterioles. Average blood pressure is 120/80. The top number represents systolic blood pressure. It is the force against the artery walls created by the contraction of the heart. The bottom number represents diastolic blood pressure. It is the resistance to blood flow caused by the smooth muscle tissue in the arteriole walls. High blood pressure is a condition when systolic pressure exceed 140 mm Hg or when diastolic pressure exceeds 90 mm Hg.

It has been estimated that 60 million Americans have hypertension. It is called the silent killer since there are no signs or symptoms. Hypertension itself is not a major killer. Complications resulting from hypertension are strokes, congestive heart disease and accelerated atherosclerosis.

CANCER

It has been estimated that 80 percent of all cancers have an environmental or lifestyle cause. Research has shown that non exercising females are at greater risk for reproductive system and breast cancer. Obesity seems to be related to cancer. Persons who get regular exercise are seldom obese. Adipose tissue is a source of estrogen. Active females tend to have less adipose tissue thus produce lower levels of estrogen, particularly more potent forms of estrogen which are related to cancer risk.

Non active people also have a higher risk for colon cancer. Inactive people are more apt to be constipated. Constipation has been associated with increased cancer risk.

Research has also shown that people who exercise tend to eat better, smoke less and consume less alcohol.

OSTEOPOROSIS

Osteoporosis is a condition where the bones become thin, porous and brittle. This is a result of a loss of mineral mass. Females have eight times the risk of developing osteoporosis than men. It is a disease that tends to occur after age 45. There are several reasons why the risk for females is greater. These include women having less bone mass than men, as well as a greater rate of bone mass loss especially following menopause.

Cigarette smoking, dietary calcium deficiency and a sedentary lifestyle have all been associated with osteoporosis.

LOW BACK PAIN

It is estimated that 75 million Americans suffer from low back pain each year. It is the cause for millions of lost work days and in excess of 10 million dollars in workman's compensation claims. It is the number one complaint treated by orthopedists and number two by internists.

There are several causes of low back pain. One cause is bone or rheumatoid disease. A second cause is forward or lateral pelvic tilt. Once cause of pelvic tilt is leg length discrepancy.

Most low back problems are the result of a lack of low back flexibility, a lack of hamstring muscle elasticity and poor abdominal strength. These problems can usually be resolved with activity which includes a good regiment of stretching exercises and abdominal exercise to increase abdominal muscular strength and endurance.

OBESITY

Obesity is one of the most common and least understood hypokinetic disorders. By itself obesity is seldom the cause of death. Considerable evidence, however, links it to coronary heart disease, hypertension, strokes, cancer, diabetes, low back pain, and many joint disorders.

Obesity is fat percentages that exceed 25 percent for males and 33 percent for females. Fat is gained when calorie intake exceeds calorie expenditure. Obesity can be corrected, in most cases, through a combination of proper diet and exercise.

Hypokinetic diseases are easier to prevent than cure. They usually result from a lack of physical activity. They can best be prevented by insuring that the human body receives regular and adequate physical exercise. In today's society it is difficult to accomplish the needed activity from one's occupation. It, therefore, requires regularly scheduled exercise at intensity and duration levels that will maintain strength and fitness and prevent excess fat accumulations. Proper diet will also be beneficial.

WORKSHEET 17–A

Chapter Seventeen—Hypokinetic Disease

True/False

1. Labor saving devices have resulted in an increase of hypokinetic disease.   1. _____
2. Most occupations require considerable physical effort.   2. _____
3. Poor eating habits have contributed to increases in hypokinetic disease.   3. _____
4. Physical activity is required to maintain strength and fitness.   4. _____
5. Hypokinetic diseases are the major cause of death today.   5. _____
6. Hypokinetic diseases are caused by a virus.   6. _____
7. Low back pain is one example of hypokinetic disease.   7. _____
8. Cardiovascular disease is the most prevalent degenerative disease.   8. _____
9. Cardiovascular disease affects the heart and circulatory system.   9. _____
10. Fifty percent of the time, the first symptom of cardiovascular disease is heart attack.   10. _____
11. In most cases the cause of cardiovascular disease is unknown.   11. _____
12. One's risk of cardiovascular disease can be reduced.   12. _____
13. Coronary artery disease is characterized by reduction of artery openings.   13. _____
14. Atherosclerosis is a progressive condition.   14. _____
15. Atherosclerosis begins during childhood.   15. _____
16. Heart attack is often a result of coronary arteries blocked by plaque.   16. _____
17. Angina Pectoris means heart attack.   17. _____
18. Angina Pectoris is caused by inadequate oxygen supply to heart muscle.   18. _____
19. Angina Pectoris most often occurs during sleep.   19. _____
20. Myocardial Infarction means heart attack.   20. _____
21. In myocardial infarction blood flow is terminated.   21. _____
22. Myocardial Infarction is an irreversible injury.   22. _____
23. Risk factors are the cause of heart attacks.   23. _____
24. Family history is an unchangeable risk factor.   24. _____
25. Hypertension is a changeable risk factor.   25. _____
26. Lack of physical activity is a risk factor.   26. _____
27. Pain that spreads to the shoulder, arms and neck are sign of heart attack.   27. _____
28. Stroke effects the brain.   28. _____
29. There are five basic causes of stroke.   29. _____
30. Thrombus is a stroke where a cerebral blood vessel burst.   30. _____
31. An aneurysm is a weak spot in an artery.   31. _____
32. Stroke can cause speech impediments.   32. _____
33. Unexplained dizziness, unsteadiness or sudden falls are signs of a stroke.   33. _____
34. Hypertension is high blood pressure.   34. _____
35. Average blood pressure is 130/90.   35. _____
36. Blood pressure is the force exerted against the artery walls.   36. _____
37. In a blood pressure of 110/70, 110 is diastolic blood pressure.   37. _____
38. Hypertension is a condition when the systolic blood pressure exceeds 140 mm Hg.   38. _____
39. Hypertension is called the silent killer.   39. _____

40. Strokes often occur as a result of high blood pressure.   40. _____

41. Eighty percent of all cancers are estimated to have environmental or lifestyle causes.   41. _____

42. Non active people have a higher risk of colon caner.   42. _____

43. Active females have a higher risk of breast cancer.   43. _____

44. Osteoporosis is a condition that effects the blood vessels.   44. _____

45. Osteoporosis results from a loss of mineral mass.   45. _____

46. It is estimated that 75 million Americans suffer low back pain.   46. _____

47. Poor abdominal strength is a cause of low back pain.   47. _____

48. Obesity is closely linked to many other hypokinetic diseases.   48. _____

49. Obesity results when calorie expenditure exceeds calorie intake.   49. _____

50. Regular exercise can reduce one's risk of hypokinetic diseases.   50. _____

51. Most occupations require little physical effort.   51. _____

52. Forty percent of those suffering heart attack die within 24 hours.   52. _____

53. Hypokinetic diseases are related or caused by a lack of physical activity.   53. _____

54. Osteoporosis and cancer are classified as hypokinetic diseases.   54. _____

55. Coronary arteries supply blood to the heart muscle.   55. _____

56. Atherosclerosis lesions are composed of lipids, blood cells and calcium.   56. _____

57. Angina Pectoris means chest pain.   57. _____

58. Increased age and being male increases one's risk of cardiovascular disease.   58. _____

59. Obesity, cigarette smoking and stress are cardiovascular disease risk factors.   59. _____

60. Strokes are similar to coronary artery disease.   60. _____

APPENDICES

APPENDIX I

Body Composition Calculation Charts

Percent fat estimates for women, sum of triceps, iliac crest and thigh skinfolds.									
Age to the Last Year									
Sum of Skinfolds (mm)	Under 22	23 to 27	28 to 32	33 to 37	38 to 42	43 to 47	48 to 52	53 to 57	Over 58
23–25	9.7	9.9	10.2	10.4	10.7	10.9	11.2	11.4	11.7
26–28	11.0	11.2	11.5	11.7	12.0	12.3	12.5	12.7	13.0
29–31	12.3	12.5	12.8	13.0	13.3	13.5	13.8	14.0	14.3
32–34	13.6	13.8	14.0	14.3	14.5	14.8	15.0	15.3	15.5
35–37	14.8	15.0	15.3	15.5	15.8	16.0	16.3	16.5	16.8
38–40	16.0	16.3	16.5	16.7	17.0	17.2	17.5	17.7	18.0
41–43	17.2	17.4	17.7	17.9	18.2	18.4	18.7	18.9	19.2
44–46	18.3	18.6	18.8	19.1	19.3	19.6	19.8	20.1	20.3
47–49	19.5	19.7	20.0	20.2	20.5	20.7	21.0	21.2	21.5
50–52	20.6	20.8	21.1	21.3	21.6	21.8	22.1	22.3	22.6
53–55	21.7	21.9	22.1	22.4	22.6	22.9	23.1	23.4	23.6
56–58	22.7	23.0	23.2	23.4	23.7	23.9	24.2	24.4	24.7
59–61	23.7	24.0	24.2	24.5	24.7	25.0	25.2	25.5	25.7
62–64	24.7	25.0	25.2	25.5	35.7	26.0	26.7	26.4	26.7
65–67	25.7	25.9	26.2	26.4	26.7	26.9	27.2	27.4	27.7
68–70	26.6	26.9	27.1	27.4	27.6	27.9	28.1	28.4	28.6
71–73	27.5	27.8	28.0	28.3	28.5	28.8	28.0	29.3	29.5
74–76	28.4	28.7	28.9	29.2	29.4	29.7	29.9	30.2	30.4
77–79	29.3	29.5	29.8	30.0	30.3	30.5	30.8	31.0	31.3
80–82	30.1	30.4	30.6	30.9	31.1	31.4	31.6	31.9	32.1
83–85	30.9	31.2	31.4	31.7	31.9	32.2	32.4	32.7	32.9
86–88	31.7	32.0	32.2	32.5	32.7	32.9	33.2	33.4	33.7
89–91	32.5	32.7	33.0	33.2	33.5	33.7	33.9	34.2	34.4
92–94	33.2	33.4	33.7	33.9	34.2	34.4	34.7	34.9	35.2
95–97	33.9	34.1	34.4	34.6	34.9	35.1	35.4	35.6	35.9
98–100	34.6	34.8	35.1	35.3	35.5	35.8	36.0	36.3	36.5
101–103	35.3	35.4	35.7	35.9	36.2	36.4	36.7	36.9	37.2
104–106	35.8	36.1	36.3	36.6	36.8	37.1	37.3	37.5	37.8
107–109	36.4	36.7	36.9	37.1	37.4	37.6	37.9	38.1	38.4
110–112	37.0	37.2	37.5	37.7	38.0	38.2	38.5	38.7	38.9
113–115	37.5	37.8	38.0	38.2	38.5	38.7	39.0	39.2	39.5
116–118	38.0	38.3	38.5	38.8	39.0	39.3	39.5	39.7	40.0
119–121	38.5	38.7	39.0	39.2	39.5	39.7	40.0	40.2	40.5
122–124	39.0	39.2	39.4	39.7	39.9	40.2	40.4	40.7	40.9
125–127	39.4	39.6	39.9	40.1	40.4	40.6	40.9	41.1	41.4

Reprinted with permission. Pollack ML, Schmidt DH, Jackson AS. Measurement of cardio-respiratory fitness and body composition in the clinical setting. *Comp. Ther.* 1980; 6: 12-27. © American Society of Contemporary Medicine & Surgery, 4711 Golf Road, Suite 408, Skokie, IL 60076.

Percent fat estimate for men, sum of chest, abdominal and thigh skinfolds.

Age to the Last Year

Sum of Skin Folds (mm)	Under 22	23 to 27	28 to 32	33 to 37	38 to 42	43 to 47	48 to 52	53 to 57	Over 58
8–10	1.3	1.8	2.3	2.9	3.4	3.9	4.5	5.0	5.5
11–13	2.2	2.8	3.3	3.9	4.4	4.9	5.5	6.0	6.5
14–16	3.2	3.8	4.3	4.8	5.4	5.9	6.4	7.0	7.5
17–19	4.2	4.7	5.3	5.8	6.3	6.9	7.4	8.0	8.5
20–22	5.1	5.7	6.2	6.8	7.3	7.9	8.4	8.9	9.5
23–25	6.1	6.6	7.2	7.7	8.3	8.8	9.4	9.9	10.5
26–28	7.0	7.6	8.1	8.7	9.2	9.8	10.3	10.9	11.4
29–31	8.0	8.5	9.1	9.6	10.2	10.7	11.3	11.8	12.4
32–34	8.9	9.4	10.0	10.5	11.1	11.6	12.2	12.8	13.3
35–37	9.8	10.4	10.9	11.5	12.0	12.6	13.1	13.7	14.3
38–40	10.7	11.3	11.8	12.4	12.9	13.5	14.1	14.6	15.2
41–43	11.6	12.2	12.7	13.3	13.8	14.4	15.0	15.5	16.1
44–46	12.5	13.1	13.6	14.2	14.7	15.3	15.9	16.4	17.0
47–49	13.4	13.9	14.5	15.1	15.6	16.2	16.8	17.3	17.9
50–52	14.3	14.8	15.4	15.9	16.5	17.1	17.6	18.2	18.8
53–55	15.1	15.7	16.2	16.8	17.4	17.9	18.5	18.1	19.7
56–58	16.0	16.5	17.1	17.7	18.2	18.8	19.4	20.0	20.5
59–61	16.9	17.4	17.9	18.5	19.1	19.7	20.2	20.8	21.4
62–64	17.6	18.2	18.8	19.4	19.9	20.5	21.1	21.7	22.2
65–67	18.5	19.0	19.6	20.2	20.8	21.3	21.9	22.5	23.1
68–70	19.3	19.9	20.4	21.0	21.6	22.2	22.7	23.3	23.9
71–73	20.1	20.7	21.2	21.8	22.4	23.0	23.6	24.1	24.7
74–76	20.9	21.5	22.0	22.6	23.2	23.8	24.4	25.0	25.5
77–79	21.7	22.2	22.8	23.4	24.0	24.6	25.2	25.8	26.3
80–82	22.4	23.0	23.6	24.2	24.8	25.4	25.9	26.5	27.1
83–85	23.2	23.8	24.4	25.0	25.5	26.1	26.7	27.3	27.9
86–88	24.0	24.5	25.1	25.7	26.3	26.9	27.5	28.1	28.7
89–91	24.7	25.3	25.9	25.5	27.1	27.6	28.2	28.8	29.4
92–94	24.5	26.0	26.6	27.2	27.8	28.4	29.0	29.6	30.2
95–97	26.1	26.7	27.3	27.9	28.5	29.1	29.7	30.3	30.9
98–100	26.9	27.4	28.0	28.6	29.2	29.8	30.4	31.0	31.6
101–103	27.5	28.1	28.7	29.3	29.9	30.5	31.1	31.7	32.3
104–106	28.2	28.8	29.4	30.0	30.6	31.2	31.8	32.4	33.0
107–109	28.9	29.5	30.1	30.7	31.3	31.9	32.5	33.1	33.7
110–112	29.6	30.2	30.8	31.4	32.0	32.6	33.2	33.8	34.4
113–115	30.2	30.8	31.4	32.0	32.6	33.2	33.8	34.5	35.1
116–118	30.9	31.5	32.1	32.7	33.3	33.9	34.5	35.1	35.7
119–121	31.5	32.1	32.7	33.3	33.9	34.5	35.1	35.7	36.4
122–124	32.1	32.7	33.3	33.9	34.5	35.1	35.8	36.4	37.0

Reprinted with permission. Pollack ML, Schmidt DH, Jackson AS. Measurement of cardio-respiratory fitness and body composition in the clinical setting. *Comp. Ther.* 1980; 6: 12-27. © American Society of Contemporary Medicine & Surgery, 4711 Golf Road, Suite 408, Skokie, IL 60076.

APPENDIX II

Energy Cost of Activity

Activity Calories Per Minute Per Pound	
Common Activities	
Sleeping	.0066
Cooking	.021
Showering	.023
Dressing	.013
Eating	.010
Driving	.015
Reading	.008
Keyboard Typing	.012
Writing	.012
Housework	.020
Shopping	.026
Lawn Mowing	.050
Lying Down/Resting Awake	.010
TV Watching	.011
Standing Still	.012
Sports	
Archery	.030
Badminton	.044
Baseball	.031
Basketball	.067
Bowling	.044
Calisthenics	.033
Circuit Training	
HydraFitness	.065
HydraFitness PACE	.090
Universal	.052
Nautilus	.042
Free Weights	.038
Cycling	
5.5 Mph	.029
9.4 Mph	.045
13 Mph	.071
Racing	.079
Dancing	
Aerobic Low Intensity	.020
Aerobic Medium	.047
Aerobic High	.061
Fishing	.028
Football	.060
Golf	.039
Gymnastics	.030
Handball	.063
Horseback Riding	.052
Hockey, Ice	.095
Karate/Judo	.088
Jump Roping	
Low Intensity	.074
Medium	.075
High	.089
Lacrosse	.095
Racketball	.081
Rowing	
Moderate	.032
Vigorous	.090
Running	
12 Min./Mile	.060
9 Min./Mile	.088

8 Min./Mile	.095
7 Min./Mile	.104
6 Min./Mile	.115
Skating, Roller and Ice	
Low Intensity	.032
Medium	.049
High	.065
Skiing	
Cross Country	.074
Downhill	.064
Water	.052
Soccer	.059
Stairclimbing	.116
Swimming	
Backstroke	.077
Breast	.074
Butterfly	.078
Crawl	.070
Side	.055
Treading	.028
Tennis	
Low Intensity	.032
Medium	.045
High	.064
Volleyball	.023
Walking	
Normal Pace	.036
Fast	.048
Hills	.055
Wrestling	.085

ADAPTED FROM: The Relative Energy Requirements of Physical Activity in the H. B. Falls ed. by E. W. Bannister and S. R. Brown, Figures 23 and 24, Exercise Physiology, Academic Press Orlando, Fla. with permission.

The Caloric Cost of Running and Walking one mile for Men and Women, E. T. Howley and M. E. Glover, Medicine and Science in Sports and Exercise, Vol. 6 P.235, 1974, Williams and Wilkins, Baltimore, MD. with permission.

Comparison of Calorie Expenditure during Five Modes of Resistance Exercise, Data Line Vol.2 No.2, HydraFitness Industries, PO Box 599, Belton, Texas, Jerry Brentham with permission.

APPENDIX III

Nutritive Value of Selected Foods

Food	Amount	Wt.Gr.	Cal.	Gr. Pro.	Gr. Fat.	Mg. Chol.	Gr. Carb.
APPLE, RAW	1 MED.	150	80	.3	1	0	20
APPLE, JUICE	1/2 CUP	124	59	.1	0	0	15
BACON	2 SLICES	15	86	3.8	8	30	1
BLT SANDWICH	1	130	327	11.6	19	21	31
BAGEL	1	68	180	7.	1	0	35
BANANA	1	140	81	1.0	0	0	21
BEAN, GREEN	1/2 CUP	65	16	1.0	0	0	3
BEAN, LIMA	1/2	85	84	6.0	0	0	17
BEEF, CHUCK	3 OZ.	85	212	25.0	12	80	0
BEEF, CORNED	3 OZ.	85	163	21.0	10	70	0
BEEF, GROUND	3 OZ.	85	186	23.3	10	81	0
BEEF, MEATLOAF	1 PIECE	111	246	20.0	15	125	6
BEEF, SIRLOIN	3 OZ.	85	329	19.6	27	77	0
BEEF, STEAK	3 OZ.	85	403	16.7	37	66	0
BEER	12 OZ.	360	151	1.1	0	0	14
BEER, LIGHT	12 OZ.	354	96	.7	0	0	4
BOLOGNA	1 OZ.	28	86	3.4	8	15	0
BREAD, CORN	1 SLICE	78	161	5.8	6	0	23
BREAD, WHEAT	1 SLICE	25	65	2.3	1	0	12
BREAD, PUMPERNICKEL	1 SLICE	32	80	2.9	1	0	15
BREAD, RYE	1 SLICE	25	61	2.3	0	0	13
BREAD, WHITE	1 SLICE	25	68	2.2	1	0	13
BROCCOLI, COOKED	1 STALK	140	36	4.3	0	0	6
BROWNIES	1	20	95	1.3	6	18	11
BURRITO, TACO BELL	1	175	404	21	16	0	43
BUTTER	1 TSP	5	36	0	4	12	0
CAKE, CHEESE	1 PIECE	85	257	4.6	16	150	24
CAKE, CHOCOLATE	1 PIECE	69	235	3.0	8	37	40
CAKE, DEVIL'S FOOD	1 PIECE	99	365	4.5	16	68	55
CARROTS	1 7-INCH	81	30	.8	0	0	7
CAULIFLOWER	1/2 CUP	63	14	1.5	0	0	3
CELERY	8-IN STLK	40	7	.4	0	0	2
CEREAL, ALL-BRAN	1/4 CUP	21	53	3	0	0	16
CEREAL, BRAN	1/2 CUP	30	72	3.8	1	0	22
CEREAL, CHEERIOS	1 CUP	23	89	3.4	1	0	16
CEREAL, CORN FLKS	1 CUP	25	97	2	0	0	21
CEREAL, FR MIN WHT	4 BISCS	31	111	3.2	0	0	26
CEREAL, GRANOLA	1/2 CUP	57	252	5.8	10	0	38
CEREAL, GRP NUTS	1/2 CUP	57	202	6.6	0	0	47
CEREAL, LIFE	1 CUP	44	162	8.1	1	0	32
CEREAL, RSN BRAN	1 CUP	49	160	4.0	1	0	40
CEREAL, SHRD WHT	1 CUP	19	65	2.1	0	0	11
CEREAL, SPCL K	1 CUP	21	83	4.2	0	0	16
CEREAL, CRN POPS	1 CUP	28	108	1.4	0	0	26
CEREAL, FRSTD FLKS	1 CUP	35	133	1.8	0	0	32
CEREAL, TOTAL	1 CUP	33	116	3.3	1	0	26
CHEESE, AMERICAN	1 OZ.	28	100	6.0	8	27	0
CHEESE, BLEU	1 OZ.	28	100	6.0	8	25	1
CHEESE, CHEDDAR	1 OZ.	28	114	7.0	9	30	0
CHEESE, COTTAGE	1/2 CUP	105	112	14	5	15	3
CHEESE, CREAMED	1 OZ.	28	99	6	8	31	1
CHEESE, MOZZARELLA	1 OZ.	28	80	7.6	5	15	1
CHEESE, PARMESAN	1 TBSP.	5	23	2.1	2	4	0
CHEESE, SWISS	1 OZ.	28	107	8	8	26	1
CHEESEBRGR, MCD'S	1	115	321	15.2	16	40	29
CHKN SNDWCH, BRG-K	1	168	379	24	18	53	31
CHKN BRST, WTH SKN	1	98	193	29.2	8	83	0
CHKN MCNUGGETS	6	111	329	19.5	21	64	15
CHKN BRST, W/O SKN	3 OZ.	85	141	27	3	45	0

145

Food	Amount	Wt.Gr.	Cal.	Gr. Pro.	Gr. Fat.	Mg. Chol.	Gr. Carb.
CHILI CON CARNE	1 CUP.	255	339	19.1	16	28	31
CHOC FUDGE	1 OZ.	28	115	.6	3	1	21
CHOC MILK	1 OZ.	28	147	2.0	9	5	16
COCOA, HOT	1 CUP	250	218	9.1	9	33	26
COFFEE	3/4 CUP	180	1	0	0	0	0
COLE SLAW	1 CUP	120	173	1.6	17	5	6
COOKIES, CHC CHIP	2 IN DIAM	20	103	1.0	6	14	12
COOKIES, FIG BARS	4	56	210	2.0	4	27	42
COOKIES, OATMEAL	2 IN DIAM	26	122	1.5	5	1	18
COOKIES, SNDWCH	4	40	195	2.0	8	0	29
COOKIES, VAN WFRS	10	40	185	2.0	7	25	29
CORN	1 EAR	140	70	2.5	1	0	16
CORN CHIPS	1 OZ.	28	155	2.0	9	0	16
CRCKRS, CHEESE	10	10	50	1	3	6	5
CRCKRS, GRAHAM	2	14	55	1.1	1	0	10
CRCKRS, RITZ	1	3	15	.2	1	0	2
CRCKRS, SALTINES	4	11	48	1	1	0	8
CRCKRS, TRISCT.	1	5	23	.4	1	0	3
CROSST EGG SAND	1	110	315	13.	20	222	19
CUCUMBERS	9 SLICES	28	4	.3	0	0	1
DOUGHNUT, PLAIN	1	42	164	1.9	8	19	22
DRESSING, BLEU CH	1 TBSP	15	77	.7	8	4	1
DRESSING, FRENCH	1 TBSP	16	83	.1	9	0	1
DRSSNG, FR. DIET	1 TBSP	15	24	0	2	0	2
DRESSING, ITALIAN	1 TBSP	15	69	.1	9	0	2
DRSSNG, IT. DIET	1 TBSP	15	10	.1	1	0	1
DRESSING, RANCH	1 TBSP	15	54	.4	6	6	1
DRESSING, 1000 IS.	1 TBSP	15	60	.2	6	4	2
DRSSNG, DIET 1000	1 TBSP	15	25	.1	2	2	3
EGGS, HARD BOIL	1 LARGE	50	72	6.	5	250	1
EGGS, FRIED W BUT	1 LARGE	46	95	5.4	6	278	1
EGG McMUFFIN	1	138	327	18.5	15	259	31
EGG SALAD SAND.	1	111	325	10.	19	215	28
EGG SCRMBL W BUT	1	64	95	6	7	282	1
FISH SAND McDON.	1	131	402	15	23	43	34
FISH STICKS	2	56	140	12	6	52	8
FRANKFURTER	1	57	176	7	16	45	1
FRENCH TOAST	1 SLICE	65	123	4.9	4	73	15
GRAPEFRUIT	1/2 MED.	301	56	1.0	0	0	15
GRAPE JUICE	1/2 CUP	127	84	.3	0	0	21
GRAVY, BEEF	1 TBSP	17	19	.3	2	1	1
HAM	3 OZ.	85	318	20.	26	77	0
HAM, LUNCH MEAT	1 SLICE	28	37	5.5	1	13	.3
HAMB. BIG MAC	1	204	581	25.1	36	85	40
HAMB. BUN	1	40	129	3.7	2	0	23
HAMB. McDON.	1	99	257	13.	9	26	30
HAMB. 1/4 LBER	1	160	427	24.6	24	80	29
HAMB. 1/4 LBER W. CH.	1	186	525	29.6	32	107	31
HOTDOG BUN	1	40	115	3.3	2	0	20
ICE CREAM, VANILLA	1/2 CUP	67	135	3.0	7	27	14
ICE CREAM SUNDAE	1	164	357	7.	11	27	58
JAMS/PRESERVES	1 TBSP	7	18	0	0	0	5
JELLY	1 TBSP	18	49	0	0	0	13
KOOL AID SUGAR	1 CUP	240	100	0	0	0	25
LASAGNA	1 PIECE	220	357	23.6	18	50	27
LEMONADE	12 OZ.	340	137	.2	0	0	36
LETTUCE	1 CUP	75	10	.7	0	0	2
LOBSTER	1 CUP	145	138	27	2	293	0
M&M PLAIN	1 OZ.	28	140	1.9	6	0	19
M&M W PEANUTS	1 OZ.	28	145	3.2	7	0	17
MACARONI	1/2 CUP	70	78	2.4	0	0	16
MAC & CHEESE	1/2 CUP	100	215	8.2	11	21	20
MARGARINE	1 TBSP	5	34	0	4	2	0
MAYONNAISE	1 TBSP	5	36	0	4	3	0

Food	Amount	Wt.Gr.	Cal.	Gr. Pro.	Gr. Fat.	Mg. Chol.	Gr. Carb.
MILK, CHOC.	1 CUP	250	180	8	5	17	26
MILK, 2 %	1 CUP	246	145	10	5	5	15
MILK SHAKE CHOC.	10 OZ.	340	433	11.5	13	45	70
MILK SHAKE VAN.	10 OZ.	289	323	10	8	29	52
MILK, SKIM	1 CUP	245	88	9	0	5	12
MILK, WHOLE	1 CUP	244	159	9	9	34	12
MUFFIN, BLUEBERRY	1	45	135	3	5	19	20
MUFFIN, BRAN	1	45	125	3	6	24	19
MUFFIN, ENGLISH	1	57	140	4.5	1	0	26
NOODLES, EGG	1/2 CUP	80	100	3.3	1	0	19
OIL, CORN	1 TBSP	15	125	0	14	0	0
OIL, OLIVE	1 TBSP	15	125	0	14	0	0
ONIONS	1/2 CUP	105	31	1.3	0	0	7
ORANGE JUICE FR.	1/2 CUP	125	61	.9	0	0	15
ORANGE	1	45	90	5	5	35	5
PANCAKES	1 MED.	73	169	5.2	5	36	25
PANCAKES W SYRUP	1 LARGE	100	250	4.	5	24	47
PEACHES	1 MED.	175	58	.9	0	0	15
PEANUT BUTTER	2 TBSP	32	188	8.	16	0	6
PB & JELLY SAND.	1	100	340	11.4	14	0	45
PEANUTS	1 OZ.	28	166	7.	14	0	5
PEARS	1	180	100	1.1	1	0	25
PEAS	1/2 CUP	80	55	4.1	0	0	10
PEPPERS	1 MED.	200	36	2.	0	0	8
PICKLES, DILL	4 MED.	135	15	.9	0	0	3
PIE, APPLE	1 31/2 IN	118	302	2.6	13	120	45
PIE, BLUEBERRY	1 31/2 IN	158	380	4	17	0	55
PIE, CHOC CREAM	1 31/2 IN	175	311	7.4	13	15	42
PIE, PECAN	1 31/2 IN	138	583	6.3	24	13	92
PIE, PUMPKIN	1 31/2 IN	114	241	4.6	13	70	28
PINEAPPLE, RAW	1/2 CUP	78	41	.3	0	0	11
PIZZA, CHEESE	1/2 10 IN		560	34	14	110	71
POPCORN	1 CUP	11	55	.9	3	0	6
PORK, SAUSAGE	1 SMALL	17	72	2.8	6	13	1
POTATO, AU GRATIN	1 CUP	245	228	5.6	10	12	32
POTATO, BAKED	1 MEDIUM	202	145	4	0	0	33
POTATO CHIPS	10	20	114	1.1	8	0	10
POTATO, FR FRIED	10	78	214	3.4	10	0	28
POTATOES, MASHED	1/2 CUP	105	69	2.2	1	8	14
POTATO SALAD	1/2 CUP	125	179	3.4	10	85	14
PRETZELS	1 OZ.	28	113	2.8	1	0	23
PUDDING, CHOC	5 OZ.	142	205	3	11	1	30
RAISINS	1 OZ.	28	82	.7	0	0	22
RASPBERRIES	1 CUP	123	60	1.1	1	0	14
RICE, WHITE	1/2 CUP	103	113	2.1	0	0	25
RICE, WILD	1/2 CUP	100	92	3.6	0	0	19
SALAD, CHEF	1 MED	273	178	17	9	103	7
SALAD, TUNA	1 CUP	205	375	33	19	80	19
SALAMI	1 OZ.	28	128	7	11	24	0
SHRIMP, FRIED	3 OZ.	85	200	16	10	168	11
SHRIMP, BOILED	3 OZ.	85	99	18	1	128	1
SODA, COLA	12 OZ.	369	144	0	0	0	37
SODA, DIET COLA	12 OZ.	340	2	.1	0	0	0
SODA, GINGER ALE	12 OZ.	366	113	0	0	0	29
SODA, LEMON/LIME	12 OZ.	340	138	0	0	0	35
SODA, ROOT BEER	12 OZ.	340	140	0	0	0	36
SOUP, CHKN NOODLE	1 CUP	241	75	4.0	2	7	9
SOUP, MUSHROOM	1 CUP	245	216	7	14	15	16
SOUP, MINNESTRONE	1 CUP	241	80	4.3	3	2	11
SOUP, SPLT PEA	1 CUP	245	145	9	3	0	21
SOUP, TOMATO	1 CUP	245	88	2	3	0	16
SOUP, VEG BEEF	1 CUP	245	78	5	2	0	10
SOUR CREAM	1 TBSP	14	30	.4	3	6	1
SPAGHETTI/SAUCE	1 CUP	250	260	8.8	9	10	37

Food	Amount	Wt.Gr.	Cal.	Gr. Pro.	Gr. Fat.	Mg. Chol.	Gr. Carb.
SPAGHETTI, PLAIN	1 CUP	140	155	5	1	0	32
SPAGHETTI, MTBLS	1 CUP	248	332	18.6	11.7	75	39
STRAWBERRIES	1 CUP	149	55	1	1	0	13
SUGAR, BROWN	1 TSP	5	17	0	0	0	5
SUGAR, WHITE	1 TSP	4	15	0	0	0	4
SWEET POTATO	1 MED	146	161	2.4	1	0	37
SYRUP, MAPLE	1 TBSP	20	50	0	0	0	13
TACO, TACO BELL	1	83	186	15	8	0	14
TARTAR SAUCE	1 TBSP	14	74	.2	8	4	1
TEA	1/4 CUP	180	0	0	0	0	0
TOMATO JUICE	1 CUP	244	42	1.9	0	0	10
TOMATO, CATSUP	1 TBSP	15	16	.3	0	0	4
TOMATO, RAW	3 1/2 OZ	100	20	1	0	0	4
TORTILLA CHIPS	1 OZ.	28	139	2.2	8	0	17
TUNA, CAN OIL	3 OZ.	85	165	25	7	60	0
TUNA, CAN WATER	3 OZ.	99	126	27.7	1	55	0
TURKEY, ROAST	3 OZ.	85	162	27	5	73	0
VEGETABLES, MIX	1 CUP	182	116	5.8	0	0	24
WAFFLES	1	75	205	6.9	8	59	27
WATERMELON	1 CUP	160	42	.8	0	0	10
WHISKEY	1 OZ.	42	110	0	0	0	0
WHOPPER, BK	1	270	614	27	36	90	45
WHOPPER/CHS, BK	1	294	706	32	44	115	47
WINE	3 1/2 OZ.	102	87	.1	0	0	4
YOGURT, FRUIT	1 CUP	227	231	9.9	2	10	43
YOGURT, PLAIN	1 CUP	226	113	7.7	4	15	12

Adapted from "Nutritive Value of American Foods in Common Units", Agriculture Handbook No. 456, US Department of Agriculture, Washington, DC 1988.

APPENDIX IV

Human Dimension Profile—Males Under 30

Percentile	Height (In.)	Weight (lbs)	Body Fat (%)	Forearm (cm)	Biceps (cm)	Chest (cm	Waist (cm)	Thigh (cm)	Calf (cm)
99	77.5	123.7	5.7	33.4	40.6	125.6	61.1	67.0	44.3
95	74.4	134.8	8.4	32.1	38.4	111.5	64.4	59.0	41.5
90	73.9	142.3	9.6	31.3	37.2	106.8	67.1	57.1	40.3
85	73.4	148.7	10.8	30.9	36.4	104.3	68.5	55.9	39.7
80	72.9	154.	11.7	30.6	35.7	102.7	70.0	54.8	39.0
75	72.4	157.3	12.4	30.2	35.1	101.6	71.4	54.0	38.5
70	72.	160.6	13.1	29.9	34.7	100.5	72.6	53.2	38.1
65	71.6	163.8	13.8	29.6	34.5	99.4	73.5	52.4	37.8
60	71.2	167.1	14.5	29.3	33.9	98.3	74.4	51.8	37.4
55	70.8	170.4	15.1	29.0	33.5	97.3	75.3	51.3	37.0
50	70.4	173.7	15.8	28.8	33.1	96.3	76.3	50.8	36.6
45	70.	177.	16.4	28.5	32.7	95.3	77.2	50.4	36.3
40	69.6	180.4	17.1	28.3	32.3	94.3	78.4	49.9	35.9
35	69.2	183.7	17.7	28.0	31.9	93.3	79.8	49.5	35.6
30	68.8	187.6	18.7	27.6	31.4	92.3	81.2	49.0	35.2
25	68.4	191.8	19.7	27.3	30.6	91.3	82.6	48.4	34.7
20	68.1	195.9	20.8	26.9	29.9	90.3	85.0	47.8	34.1
15	67.5	200.1	22.5	25.7	28.8	89.4	87.8	47.1	33.5
10	66.8	209.1	24.4	24.4	27.7	88.1	92.0	46.5	32.6
5	66.1	224.4	26.7	23.5	26.5	85.6	98.0	45.3	31.0
1	63.9	241.4	31.	22.9	24.9	83.6	113.2	41.5	29.8

APPENDIX V

Human Dimension Profile—Females Under 30

Percentile	Height (in.)	Weight (lbs.)	Body Fat (%)	Forearm (cm)	Biceps (cm)	Chest (cm)	Waist (cm)	Thigh (cm)	Calf (cm)
99	70.22	97.68	13.8	26.8	36.9	106.7	97.5	65.6	40.3
95	68.87	102.4	15.	26.2	32.4	98.5	81.4	59.7	39.2
90	67.95	108.3	16.5	25.9	30.6	96.7	78.4	58.1	38.4
85	67.33	111.8	17.6	25.5	29.7	95.6	76.8	57.0	37.8
80	67.00	114.	18.3	25.3	29.3	94.5	75.8	56.2	37.3
75	66.67	116.2	19.	25.2	28.9	93.3	74.8	55.5	37.
70	66.35	118.3	19.7	25.0	28.4	92.	73.8	54.9	36.7
65	66.02	120.5	20.4	24.6	28.0	90.7	72.9	54.5	36.4
60	65.69	122.7	21.1	24.1	27.7	89.8	72.1	54.1	36.1
55	65.36	124.9	21.8	23.8	27.4	88.8	71.3	53.6	35.7
50	65.02	127.3	22.5	23.5	27.1	87.9	70.5	53.2	35.1
45	64.68	129.7	23.	23.3	26.8	87.1	69.8	52.8	34.5
40	64.35	132.1	23.8	23.1	26.4	86.4	69.	52.2	34.
35	64.01	134.5	24.7	23.	26.1	85.8	68.1	51.5	33.7
30	63.67	136.9	25.8	22.8	25.7	85.1	67.3	50.8	33.3
25	63.27	140.3	26.9	22.	25.3	84.5	66.4	50.	32.9
20	62.80	145.5	28.2	21.6	24.9	83.8	65.5	49.1	32.3
15	62.32	150.8	30.1	21.2	24.4	82.3	64.6	48.2	31.5
10	61.85	160.	33.3	20.6	23.7	80.8	62.6	47.1	30.8
5	61.04	178.8	36.8	20.3	22.9	76.5	60.5	45.9	30.1
1	59.58	206.6	41.3	20.	21.7	74.1	56.9	43.8	26.

Muscular Strength Profile — Males 17-19 Years
Hydrafitness WeightTraining Equipment

Percentile	Bench Press	Protraction	Squat	Overhead Press	Lat. Pull	Upright Row
1	98	135	338	84	151	108
5	126	164	415	121	187	130
10	147	180	469	135	207	143
15	156	189	515	143	221	151
20	165	195	557	148	232	158
25	173	201	580	154	239	163
30	180	207	604	159	246	168
35	185	213	628	165	253	173
40	190	220	648	171	261	178
45	196	226	667	176	269	182
50	201	232	686	182	277	185
55	207	238	705	188	285	189
60	214	243	728	193	293	192
65	221	248	759	199	300	196
70	228	254	790	205	308	200
75	236	259	813	211	315	207
80	247	270	834	218	323	214
85	259	281	855	225	336	222
90	275	295	876	241	357	233
95	298	309	925	260	374	259
99	343	349	1012	282	425	289
Mean	207.5	236.5	686.2	184.3	279.1	192.5

Percentile	Triceps Extension	Right Biceps	Left Biceps	Right Triceps	Left Triceps
1	84	40	34	30	30
5	100	41	36	35	32
10	106	42	38	41	35
15	113	43	39	45	38
20	120	44	41	46	40
25	122	45	42	47	42
30	125	47	44	48	43
35	128	49	47	49	45
40	130	52	49	52	46
45	133	55	50	54	48
50	136	56	51	55	49
55	138	56	52	56	51
60	142	57	52	57	54
65	146	58	57	58	55
70	150	59	59	59	56
75	154	61	60	60	57
80	159	65	62	61	59
85	165	66	64	63	60
90	172	68	66	64	62
95	178	71	68	68	66
99	263	88	71	78	78
Mean	142.7	56.7	52.1	55.1	51.3

Percentile	Right Grip Strength	Left Grip Strength
1	96.3	77.6
5	96.9	93.6
10	105.3	103.0
15	110.9	106.5
20	115.0	110.0
25	119.1	113.4
30	122.1	116.7
35	124.3	119.0
40	126.6	121.3
45	128.8	123.6
50	131.1	125.9
55	133.3	128.2
60	136.1	130.5
65	139.0	133.5
70	141.8	136.4
75	144.6	139.6
80	148.6	142.4
85	153.5	146.1
90	158.7	151.9
95	168.3	157.8
99	189.5	175.6
Mean	132.1	125.9

APPENDIX VII

Muscular Strength Profile — Males 20-29 Years
Hydrafitness Weight Training Equipment

Percentile	Bench Press	Protraction	Squat	Overhead Press	Lat Pull	Upright Row
1	96	111	328	83	171	98
5	142	154	454	122	195	123
10	154	175	513	140	217	140
15	165	193	551	149	236	159
20	176	200	580	155	244	165
25	183	208	596	161	250	171
30	188	216	611	167	257	177
35	194	224	626	173	263	181
40	199	230	642	178	269	184
45	205	236	657	182	279	188
50	210	242	675	187	292	192
55	217	248	694	192	305	196
60	224	254	714	197	312	200
65	231	262	733	203	319	205
70	239	269	753	212	325	209
75	246	277	778	221	331	214
80	258	285	802	232	337	220
85	271	297	827	245	349	227
90	285	314	862	262	372	236
95	310	339	904	286	406	248
99	366	387	1045	326	462	265
Mean	216.8	245.5	689.1	194.4	294.0	190.9

Percentile	Triceps Extension	Right Biceps	Left Biceps	Right Triceps	Left Triceps
1	75	9	8	39	34
5	91	20	20	41	37
10	102	25	26	43	41
15	110	28	30	44	44
20	115	31	33	48	45
25	119	34	35	48	46
30	122	36	38	49	47
35	126	40	41	50	47
40	129	45	44	51	48
45	134	47	46	53	48
50	138	49	48	54	49
55	142	50	49	55	49
60	146	52	51	57	50
65	149	53	53	58	53
70	153	55	55	59	54
75	156	57	57	61	54
80	159	59	58	63	55
85	176	61	60	65	56
90	185	65	66	67	56
95	202	73	73	68	58
99	216	83	82	69	65
Mean	142.4	46.5	46.6	54.7	49.7

Percentile	Right Grip Strength	Left Grip Strength
1	96.3	77.6
5	96.9	93.6
10	105.3	103.0
15	110.9	106.5
20	115.0	110.0
25	119.1	113.4
30	122.1	116.7
35	124.3	119.0
40	126.6	121.3
45	128.8	123.6
50	131.1	125.9
55	133.3	128.2
60	136.1	130.5
65	139.0	133.5
70	141.8	136.4
75	144.6	139.6
80	148.6	142.4
85	153.5	146.1
90	158.7	151.9
95	168.3	157.8
99	189.5	175.6
Mean	132.1	125.9

APPENDIX VIII
Muscular Strength Profile — Males 30-39 Years
Hydrafitness Weight Training Equipment

Percentile	Bench Press	Protraction	Squat	Overhead Press	Lat Pull	Upright Row
1	96	86	281	90	140	130
5	120	131	309	92	143	133
10	135	147	344	94	147	135
15	141	154	379	96	151	138
20	147	159	410	98	155	141
25	154	165	433	100	159	144
30	164	173	457	102	236	147
35	174	180	480	104	238	149
40	177	191	503	106	240	150
45	180	199	526	108	242	151
50	183	206	592	110	244	152
55	186	213	609	114	246	153
60	189	219	627	116	248	155
65	192	226	644	118	250	159
70	198	233	668	146	252	160
75	213	239	703	148	254	162
80	228	288	738	150	314	165
85	241	296	868	152	318	167
90	323	304	903	153	322	168
95	353	336	1002	154	326	169
99	377	342	1030	165	329	171
Mean	188.4	208.2	577.9	118.3	241.2	151.6

Percentile	Triceps Extension
1	80
5	81
10	83
15	86
20	87
25	90
30	92
35	95
40	98
45	102
50	109
55	119
60	129
65	135
70	143
75	144
80	145
85	146
90	147
95	148
99	149
Mean	110.0

APPENDIX IX
Muscular Strength Profile — Females 17-19 Years
Hydrafitness Weight Training Equipment

Percentile	Bench Press	Protraction	Squat	Overhead Press	Lat Pull	Upright Row
1	44	90	205	45	99	62
5	55	101	255	48	120	71
10	60	107	279	51	130	78
15	65	112	297	55	134	80
20	69	117	305	59	137	82
25	72	120	314	63	141	84
30	75	123	322	67	144	85
35	78	126	331	69	148	87
40	81	128	338	72	152	90
45	84	131	358	75	154	92
50	87	135	381	78	157	94
55	90	139	396	81	160	97
60	93	143	407	84	163	100
65	96	147	417	87	166	103
70	100	150	428	90	168	108
75	103	153	440	93	171	112
80	106	156	472	96	174	116
85	112	159	498	101	181	120
90	118	163	520	108	193	126
95	131	180	553	120	213	135
99	156	201	610	140	256	145
Mean	89.4	137.3	383.9	81.4	160.0	99.0

Percentile	Triceps Extension	Right Biceps	Left Biceps	Right Triceps	Left Triceps
1	52	3	4	20	20
5	61	4	4	21	20
10	64	6	5	23	21
15	67	7	6	24	21
20	70	8	7	25	23
25	73	9	8	26	24
30	76	9	9	26	25
35	79	10	10	27	25
40	81	11	11	28	25
45	84	12	12	28	26
50	86	13	12	31	26
55	88	14	14	31	29
60	91	15	15	32	30
65	93	16	16	32	31
70	96	17	17	33	32
75	98	19	20	35	32
80	101	22	21	37	34
85	104	26	23	38	37
90	108	28	26	39	38
95	115	32	30	40	40
99	135	43	44	41	41
Mean	90.2	15.1	14.8	30.7	28.8

Percentile	Right Grip Strength	Left Grip Strength
1	38.5	37.5
5	49.8	45.2
10	55.6	50.7
15	59.8	55.5
20	63.3	59.5
25	66.1	62.7
30	68.9	64.4
35	71.6	66.0
40	73.1	67.7
45	74.6	69.3
50	76.1	71.1
55	77.6	73.2
60	79.1	75.3
65	80.6	77.3
70	82.6	79.4
75	85.1	81.5
80	87.6	83.6
85	90.1	85.7
90	96.8	88.4
95	105.3	93.2
99	118.7	103.2
Mean	76.2	71.3

APPENDIX X
Muscular Strength Profile — Females 20-29 Years
Hydrafitness Weight Training Equipment

Percentile	Bench Press	Protraction	Squat	Overhead Press	Lat Pull	Upright Row
1	39	56	119	50	73	58
5	52	78	176	54	98	69
10	62	96	232	59	113	75
15	68	103	269	64	125	78
20	71	110	284	68	132	81
25	74	115	299	72	139	84
30	78	120	314	76	144	87
35	81	124	330	80	147	90
40	86	128	348	84	151	93
45	92	131	366	88	154	96
50	97	134	383	92	157	99
55	99	138	396	96	161	102
60	102	141	407	100	166	104
65	105	146	418	105	173	107
70	108	150	430	109	179	110
75	111	154	441	115	188	114
80	115	159	456	122	197	119
85	122	163	482	130	207	123
90	129	168	508	146	217	128
95	159	183	583	165	235	133
99	181	196	633	187	254	161
Mean	97.2	136.5	380.4	98.3	163.3	101.1

Percentile	Triceps Extension	Right Biceps	Left Biceps	Right Triceps	Left Triceps
1	62	17	15	16	14
5	69	17	15	18	16
10	71	18	16	24	20
15	74	20	17	24	20
20	76	21	17	25	21
25	78	22	18	25	22
30	80	22	18	26	22
35	82	23	19	26	23
40	83	23	20	27	24
45	85	24	21	27	24
50	86	24	21	28	25
55	88	24	21	29	25
60	89	25	22	30	26
65	91	25	22	30	27
70	95	26	23	31	31
75	102	28	24	32	33
80	109	29	24	33	34
85	112	30	28	40	35
90	115	34	29	41	39
95	127	38	33	42	40
99	137	39	34	44	41
Mean	91.2	25.6	22.3	29.6	27.5

Percentile	Right Grip Strength	Left Grip Strength
1	38.5	37.5
5	49.8	45.2
10	55.6	50.7
15	59.8	55.5
20	63.3	59.5
25	66.1	62.7
30	68.9	64.4
35	71.6	66.0
40	73.1	67.7
45	74.6	69.3
50	76.1	71.1
55	77.6	73.2
60	79.1	75.3
65	80.6	77.3
70	82.6	79.4
75	85.1	81.5
80	87.6	83.6
85	90.1	85.7
90	96.8	88.4
95	105.3	93.2
99	118.7	103.2
Mean	76.2	71.3

APPENDIX XI
Muscular Strength Profile — Females 30-39 Years
Hydrafitness Weight Training Equipment

Percentile	Bench Press	Protraction	Squat	Overhead Press	Lat Pull	Upright Row
1	32	71	81	55	130	70
5	40	77	109	57	132	72
10	51	86	156	58	135	74
15	57	95	186	59	137	76
20	60	104	204	59	140	78
25	64	109	221	60	143	81
30	67	113	247	60	148	82
35	70	118	275	60	153	83
40	74	123	284	61	156	85
45	77	128	293	61	158	86
50	80	133	302	69	161	88
55	84	139	311	72	164	89
60	88	145	320	72	166	91
65	92	149	340	73	169	96
70	95	153	369	74	171	115
75	99	156	388	75	174	119
80	103	161	406	80	176	123
85	110	168	423	86	195	128
90	120	172	463	87	205	132
95	130	176	531	88	239	171
99	260	179	566	89	247	178
Mean	86.9	132.3	311.2	69.7	165.5	100.7

Percentile	Triceps Extension
1	70
5	71
10	73
15	74
20	76
25	77
30	78
35	79
40	80
45	81
50	83
55	84
60	86
65	87
70	89
75	91
80	94
85	122
90	125
95	127
99	129
Mean	90.6

APPENDIX XII
Muscular Strength Profile — Females 17-19 Years
Keiser Weight Training Equipment

Percentile	Leg Extension Right	Leg Extension Left	Leg Curl Right	Leg Curl Left	Chest Press	Upper Back
1	25	41	26	26	46	41
5	38	47	34	33	50	49
10	48	54	39	36	54	57
15	53	59	42	39	56	64
20	59	64	45	44	58	72
25	65	71	47	49	59	79
30	72	77	49	50	61	83
35	76	79	52	51	63	87
40	79	81	54	53	64	92
45	82	83	55	54	65	95
50	86	84	57	55	66	98
55	89	86	58	56	67	102
60	92	88	60	58	68	106
65	95	91	61	60	70	109
70	97	100	64	62	78	113
75	100	105	67	64	79	117
80	105	108	70	69	81	120
85	109	111	78	74	83	123
90	113	114	83	77	84	126
95	123	123	88	80	89	129
99	144	155	98	99	109	160
Mean	84.2	87.4	58.6	56.6	70.1	95.8

Percentile	Low Back	Arm Curl Right	Arm Curl Left	Triceps Right	Triceps Left	Lateral Shoulder Raise
1	60	20	20	53	53	16
5	63	22	22	79	79	18
10	67	32	32	89	88	19
15	73	32	32	95	93	20
20	79	33	33	99	97	21
25	81	33	34	101	99	21
30	83	34	35	103	102	22
35	85	35	35	105	104	23
40	89	38	36	107	106	24
45	96	38	37	110	108	29
50	99	39	38	116	116	31
55	102	39	38	121	125	32
60	105	40	39	135	131	34
65	108	40	39	139	137	35
70	110	41	40	143	143	40
75	113	44	40	148	148	40
80	116	45	44	152	152	41
85	120	46	45	156	156	42
90	125	47	46	161	161	43
95	142	48	47	165	165	46
99	148	49	49	169	169	49
Mean	98.8	39.0	38.3	122.0	121.2	31.2

Muscular Strength Profile — Females 17-19 Years

Percentile	Military Press	Butterfly	Lateral Pull Down	Abdominals	Hip Abduction
1	21	16	40	41	37
5	28	19	41	46	55
10	35	20	42	57	73
15	36	22	43	60	78
20	37	23	45	62	79
25	38	23	47	65	80
30	39	24	49	68	82
35	41	29	55	71	83
40	42	30	56	73	84
45	43	30	57	74	85
50	45	31	58	76	88
55	46	32	59	78	90
60	47	34	65	79	93
65	48	35	65	88	95
70	49	40	66	90	98
75	50	41	67	93	101
80	55	42	68	95	105
85	56	42	69	104	110
90	57	44	82	109	114
95	59	46	87	113	117
99	68	49	89	118	119
Mean	47.6	32.4	61.5	81.0	90.3

Percentile	Hip Adduction	Squat	Leg Press Right	Leg Press Left
1	91	89	261	245
5	95	105	293	268
10	100	126	302	287
15	105	157	312	301
20	108	162	322	316
25	111	167	331	324
30	114	171	338	333
35	117	176	345	341
40	120	181	353	349
45	124	185	360	357
50	128	190	367	386
55	133	199	376	402
60	138	236	386	411
65	143	248	395	421
70	148	260	405	430
75	153	274	425	442
80	159	289	458	456
85	164	304	498	470
90	176	335	518	495
95	204	389	592	534
99	234	437	638	618
Mean	138.4	218.8	392.4	385.6

APPENDIX XIII
Muscular Strength Profile — Females 20-29 Years
Keiser Weight Training Equipment

Percentile	Leg Extension Right	Leg Extension Left	Leg Curl Right	Leg Curl Left	Chest Press	Upper Back
1	23	33	21	30	45	73
5	43	48	25	34	55	80
10	53	56	35	38	57	84
15	63	62	40	41	59	89
20	68	71	46	45	61	91
25	72	74	49	48	63	94
30	76	76	50	50	65	97
35	79	78	51	51	66	99
40	82	80	53	53	68	102
45	86	84	54	55	69	104
50	89	89	56	56	71	107
55	92	93	58	57	72	109
60	96	95	61	58	74	112
65	99	97	64	59	75	115
70	102	99	69	63	77	118
75	105	102	70	67	79	120
80	108	106	72	69	85	123
85	112	113	74	72	90	126
90	119	122	75	75	93	133
95	126	128	82	80	99	139
99	133	133	88	88	114	158
Mean	87.9	89.2	57.6	56.9	74.4	105.5

Pecentile	Low Back	Arm Curl Right	Arm Curl Left	Triceps Right	Triceps Left	Lateral Shoulder Raise
1	48	30	30	25	45	15
5	57	31	30	67	74	18
10	64	32	31	78	81	19
15	69	32	32	84	87	21
20	73	33	32	90	94	22
25	77	33	33	96	101	25
30	80	34	34	102	105	29
35	84	34	34	108	107	30
40	90	37	35	112	109	31
45	94	38	36	116	111	31
50	98	38	36	120	114	32
55	101	38	37	123	116	34
60	104	39	38	127	118	35
65	106	39	38	131	121	39
70	109	39	39	135	128	40
75	112	43	40	140	135	41
80	114	43	42	144	141	42
85	116	44	43	149	148	42
90	118	48	46	155	155	43
95	120	49	51	161	164	45
99	136	54	78	194	194	48
Mean	96.4	39.5	39.7	119.2	118.3	32.7

Muscular Strength Profile — Females 20-29 Years

Percentile	Military Press	Butterfly	Lateral Pull Down	Abdominals	Hip Abduction
1	21	11	31	46	55
5	26	17	36	52	67
10	39	19	39	55	72
15	40	21	43	57	76
20	41	23	47	60	79
25	42	24	58	65	82
30	43	25	61	69	86
35	44	26	64	72	90
40	44	28	66	75	100
45	45	29	67	76	101
50	46	30	68	78	103
55	47	32	69	79	105
60	48	34	70	81	106
65	48	36	71	82	108
70	49	38	78	84	110
75	53	40	80	85	112
80	56	42	81	87	113
85	58	44	83	89	116
90	60	47	84	101	120
95	62	52	87	108	124
99	77	77	97	117	128
Mean	48.6	33.4	65.9	78.4	98.4

Percentile	Hip Adduction	Squat	Leg Press Right	Leg Press Left
1	80	82	146	150
5	84	91	174	191
10	89	102	266	242
15	97	117	287	269
20	113	136	308	282
25	118	150	325	295
30	121	164	332	307
35	124	169	339	315
40	127	175	347	332
45	132	180	354	343
50	138	186	362	355
55	143	192	369	366
60	148	210	377	377
65	152	225	385	395
70	155	236	411	415
75	159	248	437	436
80	162	257	469	466
85	166	266	503	500
90	171	276	554	535
95	176	294	698	693
99	195	348	739	734
Mean	136.4	195.6	383.2	377.1

APPENDIX XIV
Muscular Strength Profile — Females 30-39 Years
Keiser Weight Training Equipment

	Leg Extension		Leg Curl		Chest	Upper
Percentile	Right	Left	Right	Left	Press	Back
1	40	40	45	1	40	51
5	42	44	47	6	44	58
10	45	48	49	45	55	65
15	48	60	50	48	56	88
20	60	63	51	49	57	91
25	64	66	52	50	58	94
30	75	73	52	51	58	97
35	77	77	53	52	59	99
40	79	79	54	53	63	102
45	81	81	55	54	65	105
50	83	83	59	55	66	107
55	85	86	61	58	67	109
60	87	89	63	64	68	111
65	89	92	69	65	69	113
70	100	95	70	66	71	114
75	103	99	71	67	75	116
80	105	103	71	68	77	117
85	108	106	72	69	78	119
90	112	109	74	71	85	120
95	116	121	77	73	87	131
99	123	128	79	78	89	133
Mean	82.3	83.4	60.8	57.0	68.9	105.2

	Low	Arm Curl		Triceps		Lateral Shoulder
Percentile	Back	Right	Left	Right	Left	Raise
1	60	30	30	70	70	20
5	63	30	31	73	74	20
10	74	31	32	77	79	20
15	78	31	34	87	92	21
20	80	32	35	91	97	21
25	81	34	35	101	110	22
30	82	35	36	105	115	22
35	84	35	38	106	119	23
40	85	36	38	108	124	23
45	88	38	38	110	126	24
50	92	38	39	112	128	25
55	102	39	39	122	130	25
60	105	39	39	126	133	29
65	107	39	39	129	135	30
70	108	40	40	133	137	31
75	109	44	44	134	139	32
80	111	45	45	135	142	33
85	119	45	45	136	146	33
90	121	46	46	137	151	40
95	123	49	49	138	155	48
99	124	49	49	139	159	49
Mean	95.0	39.2	40.0	115.0	124.0	28.3

Muscular Strength Profile — Females 30-39 Years

Percentile	Military Press	Butterfly	Lateral Pull Down	Abdominals	Hip Abduction
1	10	20	40	40	60
5	13	20	40	43	62
10	35	21	41	46	64
15	36	21	42	48	66
20	37	28	43	50	68
25	38	28	44	52	70
30	39	28	45	61	72
35	45	28	47	64	74
40	45	29	50	65	75
45	46	29	59	66	77
50	46	29	61	67	78
55	46	29	62	67	80
60	47	34	70	68	89
65	47	34	72	69	93
70	48	34	74	78	96
75	48	35	76	82	98
80	49	35	77	89	100
85	49	35	79	91	117
90	49	35	81	93	121
95	57	38	96	96	125
99	59	39	99	99	129
Mean	45.0	30.8	61.6	68.7	86.6

Percentile	Hip Adduction	Squat	Leg Press Right	Leg Press Left
1	70	102	252	252
5	73	110	263	262
10	77	135	277	275
15	80	140	281	279
20	85	145	286	283
25	92	151	290	287
30	110	153	295	291
35	114	156	299	295
40	118	158	304	300
45	121	161	317	328
50	128	163	331	331
55	135	166	337	334
60	138	169	344	337
65	142	174	351	340
70	146	179	358	343
75	149	185	371	346
80	153	195	385	350
85	156	239	458	437
90	160	249	466	450
95	192	259	506	487
99	198	267	517	497
Mean	125.4	173.6	351.0	349.0

APPENDIX XV
Muscular Strength Profile — Males 17-19 Years
Keiser Weight Training Equipment

Percentile	Leg Extension Right	Leg Extension Left	Leg Curl Right	Leg Curl Left	Chest Press	Upper Back
1	84	84	51	57	102	105
5	101	101	65	75	114	128
10	126	137	77	80	120	154
15	139	144	83	85	127	160
20	158	152	91	88	131	165
25	164	158	96	92	136	171
30	169	164	100	95	140	177
35	172	169	103	97	157	182
40	175	172	106	99	159	188
45	178	176	108	102	161	196
50	181	179	110	105	164	204
55	184	182	112	108	166	209
60	192	189	115	112	168	212
65	199	195	118	114	173	215
70	202	200	121	117	179	219
75	205	204	124	119	186	222
80	209	208	128	122	195	225
85	212	212	132	128	202	231
90	217	217	136	134	209	238
95	223	223	140	140	224	259
99	228	228	144	148	237	276
Mean	176.8	176.5	109.8	107.5	165.0	197.9

Percentile	Low Back	Arm Curl Right	Arm Curl Left	Triceps Right	Triceps Left	Lateral Shoulder Raise
1	85	47	47	152	161	50
5	108	54	55	162	165	51
10	124	60	59	174	171	53
15	133	63	63	187	177	55
20	140	64	65	192	196	57
25	145	66	66	197	200	58
30	147	67	67	202	204	60
35	149	69	68	207	208	63
40	152	71	70	215	212	66
45	154	73	71	224	218	69
50	156	75	72	229	226	73
55	159	77	74	234	233	76
60	168	80	77	239	237	80
65	177	84	80	244	242	88
70	181	87	83	252	247	93
75	184	90	87	260	259	98
80	188	93	91	269	275	102
85	191	96	95	277	286	106
90	200	99	98	286	294	115
95	212	103	101	299	302	126
99	234	127	137	335	335	146
Mean	161.7	78.6	77.5	232.3	229.6	84.0

Muscular Strength Profile — Males 17-19 Years

Percentile	Military Press	Butterfly	Lateral Pull Down	Abdominals	Hip Abduction
1	71	50	90	90	75
5	77	54	93	92	90
10	82	59	97	95	97
15	86	63	101	98	104
20	90	67	107	103	107
25	94	71	114	109	109
30	97	74	118	112	112
35	100	77	122	115	115
40	103	79	125	118	117
45	105	82	128	123	120
50	110	87	132	130	139
55	115	91	137	132	142
60	118	95	142	134	146
65	120	98	147	136	150
70	123	101	153	138	153
75	126	103	159	140	158
80	130	107	164	143	162
85	135	112	172	146	166
90	140	118	196	149	170
95	152	129	203	166	193
99	158	156	215	186	234
Mean	110.7	89.7	138.8	130.5	136.0

Percentile	Hip Adduction	Squat	Leg Press Right	Leg Press Left
1	128	204	317	169
5	153	224	348	311
10	170	249	380	360
15	177	274	406	391
20	184	323	439	416
25	191	341	496	440
30	199	352	522	480
35	207	362	546	525
40	216	373	555	538
45	222	385	563	550
50	228	398	572	562
55	234	410	580	574
60	240	423	589	586
65	254	438	597	599
70	265	453	667	645
75	271	471	693	681
80	277	496	719	697
85	283	565	744	713
90	318	590	770	730
95	339	615	823	746
99	355	635	884	880
Mean	234.5	409.4	581.5	554.0

APPENDIX XVI
Muscular Strength Profile — Males 20-29 Years
Keiser Weight Training Equipment

Percentile	Leg Extension Right	Leg Extension Left	Leg Curl Right	Leg Curl Left	Chest Press	Upper Back
1	78	78	49	56	93	61
5	99	95	62	63	100	119
10	115	113	76	74	108	132
15	123	128	81	80	114	144
20	131	134	84	85	119	154
25	139	140	87	89	124	163
30	146	146	90	92	129	169
35	153	151	94	95	135	175
40	160	156	98	98	140	180
45	167	161	102	100	160	185
50	174	170	105	102	164	191
55	180	180	108	104	168	196
60	184	184	111	106	171	200
65	188	189	114	108	176	205
70	192	194	117	110	181	210
75	196	199	120	115	186	215
80	202	204	124	120	191	223
85	208	210	131	127	203	230
90	215	217	139	135	222	237
95	226	227	144	144	241	256
99	243	243	151	156	256	282
Mean	167.4	167.2	105.4	103.6	161.6	190.6

Percentile	Low Back	Arm Curl Right	Arm Curl Left	Triceps Right	Triceps Left	Lateral Shoulder Raise
1	83	47	47	152	161	50
5	97	54	55	162	165	51
10	109	60	59	174	171	53
15	127	63	63	187	177	55
20	135	64	65	192	196	56
25	142	66	66	197	200	58
30	145	67	67	202	204	60
35	148	69	68	207	208	62
40	150	71	70	215	212	64
45	153	73	71	224	218	66
50	155	75	72	229	226	68
55	158	77	74	234	233	71
60	162	80	77	239	237	75
65	171	84	80	244	242	79
70	178	87	83	252	247	89
75	183	90	87	260	259	95
80	187	93	91	269	275	101
85	192	96	95	277	286	104
90	201	99	98	286	294	108
95	213	103	101	299	302	123
99	232	127	137	335	335	145
Mean	159.2	78.6	77.5	232.3	229.6	80.8

Muscular Strength Profile — Males 20-29 Years

Percentile	Military Press	Butterfly	Lateral Pull Down	Abdominals	Hip Abduction
1	61	51	58	52	44
5	67	55	77	60	66
10	72	60	92	89	86
15	76	63	99	95	95
20	80	66	105	99	101
25	83	69	107	103	105
30	86	72	110	107	108
35	89	74	113	110	111
40	92	76	116	113	114
45	95	78	119	116	118
50	98	80	129	120	122
55	102	82	138	134	127
60	108	89	142	137	132
65	112	94	146	140	137
70	116	97	150	143	143
75	120	101	154	146	148
80	125	104	161	149	154
85	129	110	167	154	160
90	137	117	188	158	169
95	152	134	197	166	178
99	158	157	212	183	230
Mean	107.4	87.4	134.1	123.2	131.5

Percentile	Hip Adduction	Squat	Leg Press Right	Leg Press Left
1	64	125	317	169
5	121	149	348	311
10	152	187	380	360
15	167	231	406	391
20	176	251	439	416
25	182	271	496	440
30	187	299	522	480
35	193	328	546	525
40	198	345	555	538
45	204	362	563	550
50	213	380	572	562
55	224	393	580	574
60	234	406	589	586
65	244	419	597	599
70	254	434	667	645
75	264	458	693	681
80	274	481	719	697
85	285	547	744	713
90	295	571	770	730
95	324	600	823	746
99	352	632	884	880
Mean	220.0	375.3	581.5	554.0

APPENDIX XVII
Muscular Strength Profile — Males 30-39 Years
Keiser Weight Training Equipment

	Leg Extension		Leg Curl		Chest	Upper
Perentile	Right	Left	Right	Left	Press	Back
1	110	120	65	90	100	100
5	112	122	67	91	104	103
10	115	124	69	92	108	107
15	132	133	84	98	112	110
20	135	135	85	98	116	138
25	138	138	86	99	120	142
30	147	140	88	100	132	145
35	150	142	89	100	134	172
40	159	151	90	101	136	174
45	161	153	104	102	138	176
50	162	156	105	104	140	178
55	163	157	106	105	153	179
60	165	158	107	118	155	181
65	167	159	109	119	157	183
70	170	160	110	119	159	209
75	173	162	118	120	161	211
80	174	175	120	121	175	212
85	175	176	123	121	179	214
90	177	177	125	127	193	216
95	178	178	127	128	197	218
99	179	179	129	129	201	219
Mean	156.1	153.6	101.4	109.2	150.2	171.6

	Low	Arm Curl		Triceps		Lateral Shoulder
Percentile	Back	Right	Left	Right	Left	Raise
1	100	60	60	200	200	40
5	103	60	61	201	201	41
10	107	61	62	203	202	43
15	110	62	63	204	203	44
20	148	63	64	206	205	46
25	150	63	65	236	235	48
30	151	64	66	237	235	49
35	152	65	67	237	236	57
40	153	66	68	238	236	58
45	154	69	68	238	237	60
50	156	70	69	239	237	62
55	157	71	69	239	237	69
60	158	72	70	240	238	70
65	159	72	70	240	238	72
70	174	73	71	241	239	90
75	178	74	71	241	239	90
80	181	75	72	242	240	91
85	209	87	97	255	246	92
90	212	88	98	257	247	93
95	216	89	99	258	248	94
99	219	89	99	259	249	94
Mean	160.0	72.0	73.0	236.0	234.0	67.5

Muscular Strength Profile — Males 30-39 Years

Percentile	Military Press	Butterfly	Lateral Pull Down	Abdominals	Hip Abduction
1	60	20	90	90	100
5	61	22	91	91	101
10	62	25	93	93	102
15	63	28	94	95	103
20	68	57	96	97	112
25	70	60	97	99	114
30	71	63	99	100	115
35	76	65	101	108	116
40	77	68	104	110	117
45	78	71	107	112	118
50	80	74	110	114	120
55	89	76	113	115	128
60	90	79	116	117	129
65	91	82	119	119	129
70	96	101	132	127	130
75	97	103	135	129	131
80	97	104	138	130	131
85	98	105	181	144	136
90	98	107	184	146	137
95	99	108	187	148	138
99	99	109	189	149	139
Mean	83.3	75.0	125.0	116.6	122.5

Percentile	Hip Adduction	Squat	Leg Press Right	Leg Press Left
1	171	320	321	500
5	175	323	329	501
10	180	327	339	502
15	186	330	348	503
20	225	334	358	505
25	227	338	405	506
30	228	341	415	507
35	230	346	424	508
40	232	353	434	510
45	234	360	557	511
50	236	368	567	512
55	237	375	576	513
60	239	382	586	515
65	241	389	595	516
70	245	444	605	517
75	251	452	614	518
80	256	459	624	520
85	333	533	671	685
90	339	545	681	690
95	344	552	690	695
99	348	558	698	699
Mean	245.0	400.0	514.0	540.0

Percentile	Percent Fat	Grip Strength	Hip Flexion	Sit Ups	Push Ups	Long Jump
1	39.9	83.4	10.8	9	0	37.5
5	35.7	98.5	13.4	16	0	44.9
10	32.3	108.6	14.4	19	1	48.8
15	30.4	114.1	15.3	22	2	51.4
20	28.8	119.5	15.9	24	3	53.3
25	27.7	125.0	16.5	25	4	55.2
30	26.7	128.1	16.9	26	5	56.3
35	25.8	131.0	17.3	27	6	57.4
40	24.9	134.0	17.7	28	7	58.5
45	24.1	136.9	18.0	29	8	59.5
50	23.3	139.8	18.4	30	9	60.6
55	22.6	142.8	18.8	31	10	61.8
60	21.9	146.2	19.2	32	12	63.0
65	21.3	148.9	19.6	33	13	64.2
70	20.6	153.7	20.1	34	15	65.4
75	19.8	157.4	20.5	35	16	67.0
80	18.9	161.1	21.0	37	18	68.6
85	17.9	166.9	21.6	39	19	70.2
90	16.9	175.7	22.2	41	22	72.9
95	14.8	187.5	23.4	45	28	76.3
99	12.0	211.5	25.0	52	31	83.1
Mean	24.0	141.3	18.5		11.3	60.7

Percentile	Balance	50 Yard Dash	Side Step	Right Lateral Flexion	Left Lateral Flexion	1½ Miles
1	2.5	11.1	13	7.5	6.6	26:16
5	4.2	9.9	13	7.9	7.2	22:31
10	5.3	9.3	14	8.3	7.5	21:26
15	6.8	9.0	14	8.6	8.7	20:21
20	8.3	8.8	14	8.8	8.9	19:26
25	9.5	8.7	15	9.0	9.0	18:31
30	10.5	8.5	15	9.1	9.2	17:57
35	11.6	8.3	15	9.3	9.3	17:31
40	12.9	8.2	15	9.4	9.4	17:05
45	14.7	8.0	16	9.8	9.5	16:38
50	15.5	7.9	16	10.1	9.8	16:12
55	16.6	7.7	16	10.2	10.2	15:47
60	17.6	7.6	17	10.4	10.5	15:23
65	18.3	7.4	18	10.5	10.7	14:58
70	18.5	7.3	18	10.7	10.9	14:34
75	18.7	7.1	18	10.9	11.1	14:09
80	19.0	6.9	18	11.0	11.4	13:39
85	19.2	6.7	19	11.2	11.9	13:05
90	19.5	6.5	19	11.4	12.1	12:31
95	19.7	6.3	19	11.8	12.3	11:57
99	19.9	6.1	20	12.3	12.4	10:13
Mean	14.2	7.9	16.8	10.1	10.0	16:37

APPENDIX XIX
Physical Fitness Profile — Females 20-29 Years

Percentile	Percent Fat	Grip Strength	Hip Flexion	Sit Ups	Push Ups	Long Jumps
1	43.4	89	9.2	1	0	34.3
5	36.8	105.1	12.0	11	0	43.8
10	33.5	110.4	13.7	17	1	47.4
15	31.8	117.0	14.9	19	2	50.0
20	30.2	122.0	15.5	21	3	51.2
25	28.8	125.2	16.0	23	4	52.4
30	27.5	128.4	16.5	24	5	53.6
35	26.2	131.6	16.9	25	6	54.8
40	25.1	134.8	17.4	26	7	56.0
45	24.1	138.0	17.8	28	9	57.4
50	23.1	141.6	18.2	29	10	58.8
55	22.1	145.2	18.6	30	11	60.2
60	21.3	148.8	19.0	31	12	61.6
65	20.5	152.3	19.4	32	12	63.0
70	19.7	156.3	19.8	34	14	64.6
75	18.9	160.7	20.3	35	15	66.1
80	17.9	165.2	20.8	36	16	67.7
85	17.0	169.6	21.3	38	19	69.6
90	16.0	178.9	22.0	41	20	72.4
95	15.0	196.3	22.9	44	22	75.1
99	12.0	228.9	24.5	51	29	81.3
Mean	24.2	144.2	18.0	29.1	10.3	59.3

Percentile	Balance	50 Yard Dash	Side Step	Right Lateral Flexion	Left Lateral Flexion	1½ Miles
1	1.6	12.5	10	5.8	4.2	25:19
5	3.3	10.8	11	6.8	6.8	23:44
10	4.6	9.5	12	7.6	7.1	21:19
15	5.8	9.1	13	8.1	7.4	20:34
20	7.0	9.0	13	8.6	7.7	19:42
25	7.9	8.9	14	8.8	8.1	19:13
30	9.0	8.8	14	9.0	8.3	18:47
35	10.3	8.7	15	9.2	8.7	18:29
40	12.0	8.6	15	9.4	9.3	18:12
45	13.3	8.5	15	9.6	9.5	17:55
50	14.5	8.3	15	9.9	9.7	17:38
55	15.7	8.2	15	10.1	9.8	17:17
60	17.1	8.0	16	10.3	10.0	16:48
65	18.1	7.9	17	10.6	10.1	16:20
70	18.4	7.8	17	10.8	10.3	15:55
75	18.6	7.6	18	11.0	10.4	15:33
80	18.9	7.5	19	11.3	10.6	15:12
85	19.2	7.3	19	11.5	10.8	14:51
90	19.4	7.2	20	11.7	11.0	14:19
95	19.7	6.9	21	12.5	11.6	13:10
99	19.9	6.6	21	15.6	12.7	11:58
Mean	13.5	8.4	16.2	9.9	9.3	17:46

APPENDIX XX
Physical Fitness Profile — Females 30-39 Years

Percentile	Percent Fat	Grip Strength	Hip Flexion	Sit Ups	Push Ups	Long Jump
1	45.6	57.1	8.0	0	0	28.8
5	40.3	87.1	11.5	3	0	34.3
10	37.6	100.8	13.1	7	0	40.9
15	35.6	106.9	13.9	11	1	43.3
20	33.9	113.0	14.6	13	1	45.7
25	32.1	118.7	15.3	16	2	47.9
30	30.3	123.0	15.9	18	2	49.2
35	29.0	127.3	16.4	19	2	50.5
40	27.9	131.6	17.0	21	3	51.8
45	26.8	135.9	17.6	22	3	53.1
50	25.9	139.1	17.9	23	4	54.5
55	25.1	142.4	18.3	24	4	55.8
60	24.3	145.6	18.7	25	6	57.2
65	23.5	148.8	19.0	26	7	58.6
70	22.7	152.0	19.4	28	9	59.9
75	21.6	156.7	19.8	30	10	61.4
80	20.6	163.0	20.3	31	11	63.0
85	19.5	169.3	20.9	34	12	64.6
90	18.0	177.7	21.4	36	17	66.3
95	16.5	187.3	22.7	40	26	69.7
99	13.6	214.5	25.2	48	41	90.4
Mean	27.0	137.8	17.5	23.1	7.0	54.3

Percentile	Balance	50 Yard Dash	Side Step	Right Lateral Flexion	Left Lateral Flexion	1½ Miles
1	1.3	12.2	6	4.2	5.0	24:55
5	2.6	11.5	9	6.4	6.2	23:33
10	3.5	10.1	11	7.4	7.1	21:00
15	4.3	9.9	11	8.0	7.6	20:08
20	5.3	9.8	12	8.2	8.0	19:51
25	6.4	9.6	13	8.4	8.3	19:35
30	7.5	9.5	13	8.5	8.6	19:18
35	8.5	9.3	14	8.7	8.9	19:02
40	9.3	9.2	14	8.9	9.1	18:40
45	10.1	9.1	14	9.1	9.3	18:13
50	11.5	8.9	15	9.2	9.5	17:47
55	13.0	8.8	15	9.4	9.7	17:20
60	14.1	8.8	15	9.6	9.9	16:53
65	16.2	8.7	15	9.7	10.1	16:26
70	17.9	8.6	16	9.9	10.3	15:55
75	18.3	8.5	16	10.1	10.5	15:19
80	18.7	8.4	16	10.4	10.8	14:45
85	19.0	8.2	17	10.7	11.0	14:18
90	19.3	8.0	17	11.1	11.4	13:51
95	19.6	7.5	19	12.5	11.8	13:18
99	19.9	6.9	20	13.7	14.7	12:21
Mean	12.0	9.0	14.8	9.5	9.3	17:37

APPENDIX XXI
Physical Fitness Profile — Females 40-49

Percentile	Percent Fat	Grip Strength	Hip Flexion	Sit Ups	Push Ups	Long Jump
1	44.0	88.5	8.0	0	0	30.6
5	40.8	90.7	11.8	2	0	33.0
10	38.6	93.5	12.5	4	0	35.5
15	37.3	96.3	13.2	6	0	37.5
20	36.1	108.4	13.6	8	1	39.5
25	35.0	111.1	14.1	9	1	41.5
30	33.9	113.9	14.5	10	1	43.4
35	32.8	116.7	15.0	11	1	44.8
40	31.6	119.5	15.5	15	2	45.8
45	30.5	122.3	16.0	16	2	47.0
50	29.4	125.1	16.4	17	2	47.9
55	28.3	127.8	16.7	19	2	48.6
60	27.2	130.6	17.1	20	3	49.3
65	26.0	133.4	17.4	22	4	49.9
70	24.9	136.2	17.9	24	6	50.6
75	24.1	139.8	18.3	27	8	51.3
80	23.2	148.2	18.8	29	10	52.0
85	22.2	163.0	20.1	31	13	54.4
90	20.9	170.3	20.9	34	15	57.1
95	19.3	180.8	21.4	36	17	61.3
99	17.4	187.5	21.8	38	27	71.5
Mean	29.6	128.3	16.4	18.7	4.8	46.7

Percentile	Balance	50 Yard Dash	Side Step	Right Lateral Flexion	Left Lateral Flexion	1½ Miles
1	2.1	11.4	6	5.1	5.5	26:06
5	2.7	11.3	8	5.5	5.7	24:31
10	3.5	11.2	9	5.7	6.0	22:41
15	4.2	11.1	10	5.8	6.2	22:20
20	4.9	11.0	11	6.0	6.5	21:58
25	5.6	10.9	11	6.1	6.7	21:36
30	6.4	10.8	12	6.4	6.9	20:52
35	7.2	10.7	12	6.6	7.0	19:54
40	8.4	10.7	12	7.1	7.4	19:03
45	9.7	10.6	13	7.5	8.3	18:48
50	10.8	10.0	13	7.8	8.5	18:34
55	11.7	9.9	14	8.2	8.6	18:19
60	12.6	9.8	14	8.8	8.8	18:04
65	14.3	9.1	15	9.4	8.9	17:43
70	16.7	9.1	15	9.8	9.1	17:13
75	18.0	9.0	15	10.1	9.2	16:44
80	18.5	8.9	15	10.4	9.9	15:24
85	18.9	8.9	15	10.5	10.2	14:40
90	19.2	8.8	16	10.7	10.4	14:04
95	19.6	8.7	16	10.8	10.7	13:35
99	19.9	8.6	16	10.9	10.9	13:11
Mean	11.4	10.0	13.2	8.2	8.1	18:42

APPENDIX XXII
Physical Fitness Profile — Males 17-19 Years

Percentile	Percent Fat	Grip Strength	Hip Flexion	Sit Ups	Push Ups	Long Jump
1	32.1	145.3	9.1	19	11	54.2
5	24.9	174.6	12.2	25	15	65.3
10	21.1	198.5	13.6	29	18	69.5
15	19.0	202.0	14.3	31	22	72.3
20	17.6	208.1	14.9	32	26	74.4
25	16.6	214.1	15.5	34	28	76.5
30	15.6	220.2	16.0	36	30	78.3
35	14.6	225.5	16.4	37	31	80.0
40	13.9	230.0	16.9	38	33	81.7
45	13.3	234.6	17.4	39	35	83.3
50	12.7	238.1	17.8	40	37	84.6
55	12.2	243.6	18.2	41	39	86.0
60	11.6	248.1	18.5	43	40	87.3
65	11.0	253.3	18.9	44	41	88.6
70	10.4	259.3	19.4	45	43	90.1
75	9.5	265.4	19.9	47	44	91.7
80	8.6	271.5	20.4	48	45	93.2
85	7.8	277.5	20.9	49	46	94.7
90	6.9	291.0	21.6	52	48	97.3
95	5.1	305.1	22.6	56	50	100.1
99	3.5	330.0	24.3	64	58	105.2
Mean	13.5	239.2	17.6	41.1	36.0	84.2

Percentile	Balance	50 Yard Dash	Side Step	Right Lateral Flexion	Left Lateral Flexion	1½ Miles
1	3.5	8.0	15	7.0	5.6	20:29
5	5.6	7.6	16	7.2	6.2	16:28
10	8.4	7.4	17	7.5	7.6	15:56
15	10.6	7.1	18	7.9	8.9	15:02
20	12.3	7.0	18	8.6	9.0	14:13
25	14.3	7.0	18	9.0	9.2	13:39
30	15.7	6.9	19	9.4	9.3	13:05
35	16.9	6.8	19	9.6	9.5	12:34
40	18.0	6.7	19	9.7	9.6	12:17
45	18.3	6.7	19	9.9	9.8	11:59
50	18.5	6.6	20	10.1	9.9	11:41
55	18.6	6.5	20	10.3	10.0	11:23
60	18.8	6.5	20	10.5	10.2	11:05
65	18.9	6.4	20	10.6	10.3	10:48
70	19.1	6.4	21	10.8	10.4	10:31
75	19.2	6.3	21	11.0	10.8	10:13
80	19.4	6.3	22	11.5	11.6	9:56
85	19.5	6.2	22	12.1	12.0	9:39
90	19.7	6.1	23	13.0	12.7	9:22
95	19.8	5.9	23	14.3	13.5	8:44
99	19.9	5.7	23	14.8	13.9	7:42
Mean	16.7	6.7	20.1	10.2	10.0	12:12

APPENDIX XXIII
Physical Fitness Profile — Males 20-29 Years

Percentile	Percent Fat	Grip Strength	Hip Flexion	Sit Ups	Push Ups	Long Jump
1	30.8	151.8	9.3	19	9	57.8
5	26.1	183.4	11.7	24	13	65.3
10	23.5	196.5	13.3	27	15	70.1
15	21.8	209.1	14.0	29	17	72.7
20	20.1	214.9	14.6	32	18	75.1
25	19.1	220.3	15.1	34	20	77.5
30	18.1	225.8	15.6	35	23	79.1
35	17.0	231.2	16.1	36	25	80.7
40	16.2	236.5	16.6	37	27	82.2
45	15.3	241.3	17.1	39	28	83.8
50	14.5	246.2	17.5	40	29	85.2
55	13.7	251.1	17.9	41	31	86.6
60	12.9	256.0	18.3	42	33	88.0
65	12.2	260.8	18.6	43	37	89.3
70	11.5	267.1	19.0	44	39	90.7
75	10.7	273.4	19.4	46	41	92.2
80	10.0	279.7	19.9	48	42	94.0
85	8.8	286.0	20.5	49	44	95.8
90	7.7	298.9	21.0	52	46	97.5
95	6.6	312.8	22.1	55	48	101.5
99	3.8	345.5	23.8	61	56	107.5
Mean	15.2	247.0	17.3	39.9	32.1	84.6

Percentile	Balance	50 Yard Dash	Side Step	Right Lateral Flexion	Left Lateral Flexion	1½ Miles
1	3.5	8.1	8	7.5	6.0	16:14
5	6.0	7.6	9	7.6	6.2	16:01
10	8.9	7.4	10	7.8	6.4	15:44
15	10.9	7.2	11	8.0	6.7	13:50
20	13.3	7.1	16	8.2	7.9	13:16
25	15.1	7.0	17	8.4	8.3	12:43
30	16.6	6.9	18	8.6	8.8	12:16
35	17.8	6.9	18	9.5	9.2	13:05
40	18.3	6.8	19	9.7	9.3	11:54
45	18.4	6.8	19	9.9	9.4	11:42
50	18.5	6.7	19	10.1	9.5	11:31
55	18.7	6.7	19	10.2	9.7	11:23
60	18.8	6.6	20	10.4	9.8	11:15
65	19.0	6.6	20	10.6	9.9	11:06
70	18.1	6.5	21	11.6	10.3	10:58
75	19.2	6.4	21	12.0	10.8	10:50
80	19.4	6.3	21	12.4	11.2	10:34
85	19.5	6.2	22	12.8	13.2	10:01
90	19.7	6.1	22	13.2	13.5	9:27
95	19.8	6.0	22	13.6	13.7	8:54
99	19.9	5.8	22	13.9	13.9	8:27
Mean	17.0	6.7	18.7	10.3	9.8	12:00

APPENDIX XXIV
Physical Fitness Profile — Males 30-39 Years

Percentile	Percent Fat	Grip Strength	Hip Flexion	Sit Ups	Push Ups	Long Jump
1	46.6	129.1	7.2	12	5	48.3
5	40.5	173.6	10.0	17	7	53.7
10	28.4	200.8	11.0	20	9	58.5
15	26.2	211.0	11.8	22	11	62.4
20	24.3	221.1	12.7	24	14	65.5
25	22.9	226.8	13.6	26	16	68.1
30	21.6	231.4	14.0	27	18	70.1
35	20.7	236.1	14.4	28	20	72.0
40	19.9	240.8	14.8	29	22	73.5
45	19.1	245.5	15.2	31	24	74.5
50	18.4	251.3	15.7	32	26	75.6
55	17.6	257.1	16.2	33	28	76.6
60	16.8	262.9	16.6	35	30	77.6
65	16.0	268.7	17.1	36	32	78.7
70	15.2	274.5	17.8	37	34	82.1
75	14.2	314.9	18.2	39	42	85.4
80	13.2	335.2	21.7	40	59	87.8
85	12.2	378.2	24.6	42	62	99.3
90	10.8	398.5	25.6	44	71	109.5
95	9.1	418.7	26.7	46	74	113.8
99	6.3	435.0	27.6	51	76	117.3
Mean	19.1	250.6	15.7	32.5	29.8	76.0

Percentile	Balance	50 Yard Dash	Side Step	Right Lateral Flexion	Left Lateral Flexion	1½ Miles
1	2.0	8.8	12	7.5	7.5	20:22
5	3.8	8.7	13	7.7	7.7	20:03
10	5.3	8.6	14	7.9	7.9	19:40
15	10.8	8.5	14	8.1	9.3	19:16
20	12.3	8.4	15	8.3	9.5	18:06
25	13.5	7.6	15	8.6	9.6	17:42
30	14.7	7.5	15	8.8	9.7	16:08
35	16.1	7.4	16	9.0	9.8	15:56
40	16.8	7.3	17	9.8	9.9	15:44
45	18.2	7.3	18	10.0	10.7	15:21
50	18.3	7.2	18	10.2	10.9	14:10
55	18.5	7.2	18	10.4	11.1	13:58
60	18.7	6.9	18	10.6	11.3	13:46
65	18.9	6.8	19	10.9	11.5	13:35
70	19.1	6.8	19	11.1	11.8	11:49
75	19.3	6.7	19	11.3	11.9	11:37
80	19.4	6.7	20	12.1	12.1	11:25
85	19.5	6.6	20	12.3	12.2	11:13
90	19.6	6.6	23	12.5	12.4	11:02
95	19.8	6.5	24	12.7	12.5	10:38
99	19.9	6.5	25	12.9	12.7	10:19
Mean	16.0	7.4	18.3	10.1	10.7	14:27

APPENDIX XXV
Physical Fitness Profile — Males 40-49 Years

Percentile	Percent Fat	Grip Strength	Hip Flexion	Sit Ups	Push Ups	Long Jump
1	32.7	109.0	8.7	0	2	45.4
5	31.1	179.7	9.6	2	4	47.2
10	29.5	195.4	10.6	11	6	49.4
15	28.2	205.7	11.6	14	8	51.6
20	27.1	216.0	12.1	16	11	57.4
25	25.8	220.4	12.6	18	13	58.5
30	24.4	224.4	13.1	19	15	59.6
35	23.9	228.4	13.4	20	18	60.7
40	23.4	232.4	13.7	21	19	66.6
45	23.0	236.4	14.0	22	21	68.8
50	22.5	240.4	14.3	23	22	69.6
55	21.5	246.5	14.7	23	23	70.4
60	20.2	253.1	15.1	24	24	71.1
65	19.4	259.6	15.5	25	25	71.8
70	18.6	266.2	15.9	25	26	72.6
75	17.6	273.4	16.4	26	28	78.0
80	15.7	280.6	17.1	27	29	80.2
85	14.9	287.8	17.8	29	30	81.7
90	14.1	302.7	19.3	32	55	82.8
95	13.0	320.7	21.4	35	57	83.9
99	11.8	335.1	23.0	37	59	84.7
Mean	21.8	245.1	14.7	21.8	24.0	67.6

Percentile	Balance	50 Yard Dash	Side Step	Right Lateral Flexion	Left Lateral Flexion	1½ Miles
1	3.0	8.1	9	8.0	9.0	17:56
5	3.2	8.1	9	8.0	9.0	17:52
10	3.5	8.1	10	8.0	9.2	17:47
15	3.7	8.0	10	8.2	9.3	17:42
20	4.0	7.7	11	8.2	9.4	17:37
25	4.2	7.7	13	8.4	9.4	17:31
30	4.5	7.6	14	8.4	9.5	17:26
35	4.9	7.6	14	8.5	9.9	17:21
40	5.5	7.6	15	8.6	9.9	17:17
45	6.1	7.5	15	8.8	10.0	17:11
50	7.2	7.5	15	8.9	10.0	15:23
55	11.9	7.5	18	8.9	10.1	15:10
60	13.2	7.1	18	9.0	10.1	14:57
65	13.6	7.1	18	9.1	10.2	14:41
70	14.0	7.1	18	9.3	10.2	14:15
75	14.4	7.0	19	9.5	10.3	13:49
80	14.9	6.8	19	9.7	10.3	13:23
85	18.7	6.8	19	9.8	10.4	12:57
90	19.1	6.8	19	9.9	10.4	12:30
95	19.5	6.7	19	9.9	10.5	10:30
99	19.9	6.7	19	10.0	10.5	10:09
Mean	9.8	7.4	15.8	9.0	10.0	15:27

APPENDIX XXVI
Muscular Strength Profile — Females Under 20 Years
Omni-Tron Strength Testing
Peak Force/Torque

Percentile	Bench Press	Bench Pull	Right Quad	Left Quad	Right Hamst.	Left Hamst.	Overhead Press	Lat. Pull
1	62	53	36	38	27	28	25	23
5	70	59	47	46	34	32	28	45
10	77	63	52	50	36	35	31	51
15	82	66	54	53	37	38	34	56
20	86	68	57	55	39	39	36	59
25	89	70	59	58	40	40	38	62
30	91	73	60	59	41	41	40	64
35	93	75	62	61	42	41	42	66
40	96	77	63	62	43	42	43	68
45	98	79	65	64	44	43	46	69
50	101	83	67	66	45	43	48	71
55	104	86	68	67	47	45	49	73
60	106	88	70	69	48	46	51	74
65	109	90	72	71	49	48	53	76
70	113	92	74	73	51	49	54	79
75	118	95	77	75	52	51	57	81
80	124	98	81	77	53	52	59	84
85	129	101	83	79	57	55	62	87
90	134	105	86	82	62	58	66	91
95	148	110	90	86	65	62	72	96
99	173	116	99	94	70	66	82	107
Mean	104.7	83.8	67.9	66.4	47.1	45.8	48.6	71.5

Power

Percentile	Bench Press	Bench Pull	Right Quad	Left Quad	Right Hamst.	Left Hamst.	Overhead Press	Lat. Pull
1	32	34	40	30	22	24	15	41
5	39	39	48	42	35	31	18	50
10	48	45	58	55	38	40	21	62
15	57	50	64	61	42	42	24	67
20	64	53	69	67	46	45	27	72
25	67	56	75	73	49	47	31	76
30	71	59	80	79	52	49	34	80
35	74	61	85	84	55	52	37	84
40	78	64	88	88	58	54	39	88
45	81	67	92	93	61	57	42	92
50	85	71	96	97	63	60	44	97
55	89	75	100	102	66	70	46	102
60	92	80	104	106	69	67	48	107
65	97	84	109	111	73	70	50	112
70	105	90	115	116	76	74	53	118
75	112	96	120	121	79	79	55	126
80	120	102	126	126	82	84	57	134
85	131	108	135	131	93	89	59	141
90	163	115	144	148	107	97	70	154
95	215	129	179	180	123	109	96	167
99	341	187	250	260	170	187	194	283
Mean	98.0	77.7	102.0	102.1	68.7	66.2	48.1	105.2

APPENDIX XXVII
Muscular Strength Profile — Females 20-29 Years
Omni-Tron Strength Testing
Peak Force/Torque

Percentile	Bench Press	Bench Pull	Right Quad	Left Quad	Right Hamst.	Left Hamst.	Overhead Press	Lat. Pull
1	53	46	35	31	24	24	23	36
5	71	58	45	45	29	29	27	45
10	77	65	51	51	34	34	31	55
15	82	69	56	55	37	37	35	58
20	89	72	57	57	39	38	37	61
25	93	75	59	59	40	40	39	63
30	96	78	60	61	41	41	41	65
35	98	79	61	63	42	42	43	67
40	101	81	63	65	43	43	45	69
45	103	82	64	67	44	44	47	71
50	105	84	66	69	45	45	48	72
55	108	86	68	71	46	46	50	74
60	110	88	70	73	47	47	52	76
65	113	90	72	75	49	48	54	79
70	116	92	74	77	50	50	56	81
75	121	95	78	79	52	51	57	83
80	124	99	82	81	56	53	59	90
85	128	104	86	85	59	55	63	95
90	132	111	90	89	63	57	66	99
95	137	117	94	95	67	62	69	103
99	149	125	98	100	70	69	82	110
Mean	106.1	85.9	68.6	69.6	47.1	45.7	49.5	73.8

Power

Percentile	Bench Press	Bench Pull	Right Quad	Left Quad	Right Hamst.	Left Hamst.	Overhead Press	Lat. Pull
1	33	21	34	28	23	19	11	41
5	41	35	49	44	31	29	13	51
10	51	47	59	59	37	38	16	66
15	59	52	68	69	42	43	19	74
20	62	58	72	73	46	47	22	78
25	66	61	75	78	49	50	25	82
30	70	63	79	83	52	52	28	86
35	74	66	83	87	55	54	31	90
40	78	69	88	91	58	56	34	94
45	81	72	93	95	61	58	37	98
50	86	74	98	98	64	61	40	102
55	91	77	103	102	67	63	43	106
60	96	80	108	105	69	66	46	110
65	101	82	113	109	72	69	48	114
70	106	85	118	115	74	72	51	118
75	111	89	124	123	79	76	54	128
80	121	94	132	130	87	79	56	140
85	130	98	140	139	92	83	59	154
90	142	106	149	148	97	88	62	161
95	157	118	160	161	108	99	65	170
99	267	138	179	226	120	117	91	194
Mean	93.8	75.4	100.4	102.5	66.5	62.9	44.0	107.0

APPENDIX XXVIII
Muscular Strength Profile — Females 30-39
Omni-Tron Strength Testing
Peak Force/Torque

Percentile	Bench Press	Bench Pull	Right Quad	Left Quad	Right Hamst.	Left Hamst.	Overhead Press	Lat. Pull
1	62	41	27	19	27	25	24	41
5	69	49	36	31	30	29	30	53
10	77	58	43	42	33	32	33	62
15	86	64	47	51	36	36	35	65
20	86	71	50	54	38	37	38	68
25	91	76	53	56	39	38	40	71
30	93	79	55	58	40	39	42	73
35	96	82	57	60	41	40	44	76
40	99	85	59	62	42	41	47	77
45	101	88	60	64	43	43	50	79
50	104	91	62	66	43	44	51	80
55	107	94	65	68	45	45	52	82
60	110	98	67	70	47	46	54	83
65	114	102	70	72	49	47	55	84
70	117	105	73	74	51	48	57	86
75	120	109	77	76	52	50	59	87
80	125	113	82	79	54	52	61	91
85	131	119	87	83	58	53	63	96
90	137	124	93	88	63	61	67	101
95	153	131	104	97	73	74	79	110
99	206	208	119	131	82	81	86	156
Mean	108.6	94.0	65.8	67.0	46.7	46.4	50.6	82.1

Power

Percentile	Bench Press	Bench Pull	Right Quad	Left Quad	Right Hamst.	Left Hamst.	Overhead Press	Lat. Pull
1	40	31	21	13	23	21	17	39
5	45	38	29	23	27	25	23	55
10	51	46	41	38	31	31	24	74
15	57	55	51	52	37	37	26	82
20	64	59	56	65	42	42	28	87
25	70	62	62	67	46	45	30	91
30	75	65	66	70	49	49	33	97
35	78	67	70	72	52	52	35	102
40	82	70	73	75	53	53	38	107
45	86	73	77	78	55	55	40	110
50	90	75	81	80	57	57	42	112
55	93	78	85	83	59	59	44	115
60	97	82	89	89	61	60	48	117
65	101	86	94	94	64	63	52	120
70	105	90	101	100	67	65	55	126
75	111	94	108	105	70	67	58	132
80	122	99	118	111	75	70	60	140
85	132	103	126	116	81	84	63	148
90	145	109	132	125	87	91	65	157
95	169	115	145	139	95	100	69	167
99	361	120	161	181	114	118	85	175
Mean	98.3	77.9	85.1	84.5	59.3	58.7	45.0	111.6

APPENDIX XXIX
Muscular Strength Profile — Females 40-49
Omni-Tron Strength Testing
Peak Force/Torque

Percentile	Bench Press	Bench Pull	Right Quad	Left Quad	Right Hamst.	Left Hamst.	Overhead Press	Lat. Pull
1	58	52	38	43	33	32	15	30
5	60	55	42	44	34	33	18	33
10	63	59	44	45	35	35	29	48
15	71	63	46	46	37	36	32	51
20	75	67	48	48	38	37	34	54
25	80	73	50	50	39	38	36	66
30	84	78	53	59	40	38	37	68
35	89	82	56	60	41	39	38	71
40	93	83	58	61	42	40	40	75
45	98	84	60	63	44	42	41	77
50	100	85	67	65	46	43	42	79
55	102	85	69	66	47	44	48	80
60	104	86	71	69	48	45	50	81
65	106	87	71	70	49	46	51	83
70	107	91	72	71	51	47	53	83
75	109	95	73	72	52	48	54	84
80	110	99	74	72	53	50	56	85
85	112	102	77	73	55	52	57	86
90	114	104	80	74	57	54	58	87
95	119	108	82	77	59	55	66	88
99	225	111	84	80	66	58	69	88
Mean	94.6	84.6	63.4	63.0	46.3	43.6	45.2	72.3

Power

Percentile	Bench Press	Bench Pull	Right Quad	Left Quad	Right Hamst.	Left Hamst.	Overhead Press	Lat. Pull
1	36	20	40	47	35	29	8	26
5	40	28	47	54	36	33	12	32
10	44	35	50	56	37	35	16	59
15	48	48	53	58	38	37	20	63
20	52	51	56	59	44	40	23	66
25	56	54	60	63	45	43	27	74
30	60	66	64	68	46	44	30	84
35	65	67	68	76	47	46	33	91
40	70	69	72	81	48	52	36	96
45	75	70	80	85	52	56	38	100
50	79	71	92	89	56	57	40	107
55	82	73	102	92	59	58	41	113
60	86	74	104	97	62	59	43	116
65	89	77	106	102	68	60	44	119
70	92	81	109	107	69	62	45	122
75	95	86	115	108	70	71	46	124
80	98	93	121	110	71	72	50	126
85	102	97	123	111	73	73	56	128
90	111	101	125	113	77	74	65	130
95	121	106	127	117	79	75	70	132
99	249	111	128	121	81	75	85	134
Mean	81.9	71.6	88.2	86.8	57.5	55.4	40.4	98.8

APPENDIX XXX
Muscular Strength Profile — Males Under 20 Years
Omni-Tron Strength Testing
Peak Force/Torque

Percentile	Bench Press	Bench Pull	Right Quad	Left Quad	Right Hamst.	Left Hamst.	Overhead Press	Lat. Pull
1	94	92	68	64	50	53	50	74
5	127	103	77	72	59	58	54	89
10	141	109	81	83	62	62	58	97
15	149	115	86	89	64	64	62	105
20	156	120	89	93	67	66	66	110
25	162	124	92	95	69	68	71	114
30	170	128	95	98	71	69	75	118
35	178	131	101	100	73	70	79	123
40	184	134	106	103	75	72	83	127
45	187	137	109	106	77	73	85	130
50	190	141	112	109	78	75	87	134
55	193	145	115	112	80	77	89	137
60	196	149	118	114	82	79	91	141
65	200	154	122	116	84	81	94	144
70	206	158	125	118	85	83	96	148
75	212	162	128	120	87	85	100	153
80	219	166	131	123	89	87	106	158
85	232	174	133	128	92	89	114	164
90	253	187	138	133	94	92	124	169
95	263	196	147	140	98	95	173	181
99	271	220	160	157	103	102	200	191
Mean	190.7	145.3	111.0	108.3	78.6	76.6	90.8	135.1

Power

Percentile	Bench Press	Bench Pull	Right Quad	Left Quad	Right Hamst.	Left Hamst.	Overhead Press	Lat. Pull
1	103	75	87	85	52	49	49	100
5	128	92	102	103	80	79	62	140
10	137	102	120	120	92	89	72	155
15	147	110	137	134	98	97	77	168
20	157	119	144	146	105	103	82	178
25	164	125	149	154	110	107	88	189
30	172	131	155	162	116	112	92	199
35	179	137	160	171	121	116	96	209
40	187	143	166	178	127	120	99	218
45	196	148	175	185	132	123	102	228
50	206	154	184	191	138	127	106	239
55	215	160	193	197	143	130	109	249
60	225	166	204	204	148	133	112	259
65	234	172	215	211	153	141	119	267
70	243	180	226	218	157	150	128	274
75	253	189	236	226	162	157	138	282
80	268	197	246	233	168	165	154	290
85	283	209	255	244	174	172	167	306
90	303	220	263	261	181	179	178	327
95	346	258	276	283	194	188	199	348
99	396	296	309	329	211	200	262	377
Mean	215.9	160.5	190.7	192.8	137.6	130.5	117.2	239.6

APPENDIX XXXI
Muscular Strength Profile — Males 20-29 Years
Omni-Tron Strength Testing
Peak Force/Torque

Percentile	Bench Press	Bench Pull	Right Quad	Left Quad	Right Hamst.	Left Hamst.	Overhead Press	Lat. Pull
1	92	88	65	70	44	44	39	81
5	136	103	74	79	52	49	52	91
10	152	112	81	83	57	56	62	105
15	159	116	88	88	61	60	65	112
20	167	120	95	91	64	62	68	116
25	173	124	97	94	66	65	71	120
30	177	128	100	97	68	67	75	125
35	182	132	103	100	70	69	78	130
40	186	136	105	103	72	71	81	134
45	191	140	108	105	75	73	83	138
50	195	145	111	108	77	76	86	141
55	200	149	113	112	79	78	88	144
60	204	153	116	116	81	81	91	146
65	209	157	119	120	84	83	94	149
70	214	162	123	124	86	86	97	151
75	219	167	126	127	89	88	101	155
80	227	173	131	131	92	91	104	160
85	236	179	137	136	95	96	108	164
90	247	187	144	141	100	102	114	171
95	263	203	152	152	107	111	124	181
99	298	232	162	164	115	176	180	218
Mean	197.9	148.8	112.7	111.9	78.1	78.9	88.2	139.3

Power

Percentile	Bench Press	Bench Pull	Right Quad	Left Quad	Right Hamst.	Left Hamst.	Overhead Press	Lat. Pull
1	104	77	57	85	40	55	33	111
5	136	94	89	95	61	69	53	136
10	154	101	108	107	78	77	77	157
15	169	109	123	119	87	84	87	176
20	183	116	136	129	96	91	92	188
25	195	125	146	139	102	97	97	199
30	205	133	156	151	108	102	102	210
35	215	140	166	164	114	108	107	220
40	225	146	176	177	120	115	113	229
45	236	152	184	186	127	123	118	237
50	245	157	193	194	134	130	123	255
55	255	163	201	203	141	135	128	269
60	265	167	209	213	146	140	133	282
65	275	172	218	222	152	146	140	296
70	285	177	228	232	157	151	149	296
75	296	182	241	242	163	158	158	308
80	308	191	253	252	174	165	167	320
85	319	205	265	263	185	172	176	336
90	339	224	286	278	197	187	185	356
95	391	246	309	299	217	212	213	394
99	505	290	362	354	242	238	293	455
Mean	247.1	159.0	196.9	194.7	135.8	130.7	128.4	254.3

APPENDIX XXXII
Muscular Strength Profile — Males 30-39 Years
Omni-Tron Strength Testing
Peak Force/Torque

Percentile	Bench Press	Bench Pull	Right Quad	Left Quad	Right Hamst.	Left Hamst.	Overhead Press	Lat. Pull
1	92	55	47	56	34	36	49	62
5	123	78	64	64	41	41	60	71
10	147	121	86	78	58	57	62	103
15	154	128	88	82	61	59	65	109
20	162	135	91	86	64	60	68	114
25	166	138	93	90	67	62	70	119
30	169	140	96	93	68	63	73	122
35	173	142	99	97	70	65	75	126
40	176	144	103	101	72	66	78	129
45	180	146	106	105	74	67	81	133
50	183	149	108	108	76	68	84	136
55	186	152	110	111	77	70	86	139
60	188	156	112	114	79	72	89	143
65	191	160	114	116	80	75	92	146
70	194	164	116	118	81	77	94	149
75	197	167	118	120	83	79	97	152
80	200	170	122	123	86	81	100	155
85	207	173	126	125	90	83	109	159
90	220	177	131	131	95	90	117	164
95	240	183	138	141	101	94	126	171
99	271	191	146	152	114	101	174	177
Mean	184.4	147.9	106.7	105.0	75.2	70.8	87.7	133.2

Power

Percentile	Bench Press	Bench Pull	Right Quad	Left Quad	Right Hamst.	Left Hamst.	Overhead Press	Lat. Pull
1	135	109	96	88	67	69	71	154
5	143	119	104	104	79	73	79	173
10	154	125	115	112	87	78	88	185
15	168	132	126	121	93	86	91	197
20	186	140	142	131	101	94	94	212
25	197	145	148	141	112	98	97	225
30	208	148	153	150	120	102	99	234
35	216	151	158	158	123	106	102	244
40	221	154	163	172	126	111	105	251
45	225	157	168	186	129	115	109	259
50	230	161	172	193	132	120	113	267
55	235	165	191	200	135	125	118	272
60	240	169	197	205	139	129	123	277
65	249	177	204	209	141	132	128	283
70	258	184	210	213	144	134	133	288
75	267	189	217	218	146	137	138	294
80	275	194	223	222	149	139	144	302
85	282	199	229	234	151	143	181	310
90	290	204	234	249	157	148	199	320
95	321	223	239	260	162	165	218	332
99	391	230	252	277	171	184	251	375
Mean	229.6	164.3	178.4	183.6	127.3	118.9	127.3	258.0

APPENDIX XXXIII
Muscular Strength Profile — Males 40-49
Omni-Tron Strength Testing
Peak Force/Torque

Percentile	Bench Press	Bench Pull	Right Quad	Left Quad	Right Hamst.	Left Hamst.	Overhead Press	Lat. Pull
1	140	120	84	53	52	47	50	109
5	143	121	84	56	53	49	51	111
10	146	123	85	60	55	52	52	113
15	157	124	86	71	57	59	53	114
20	160	126	87	73	59	60	55	115
25	162	136	88	75	61	61	56	116
30	163	139	89	77	62	63	57	117
35	165	142	97	80	63	64	58	119
40	166	144	99	84	64	65	60	121
45	167	145	102	88	69	67	61	123
50	168	147	103	92	71	68	64	125
55	169	149	105	96	73	69	66	127
60	187	152	106	99	75	77	75	142
65	190	155	107	103	77	80	77	143
70	194	158	133	125	87	82	90	144
75	197	161	135	129	88	85	92	146
80	200	165	136	132	89	88	93	147
85	204	168	137	134	90	90	94	149
90	207	186	139	136	92	98	101	151
95	210	189	142	138	94	101	104	153
99	213	192	144	139	95	103	106	155
Mean	178.0	149.1	108.4	98.4	73.8	72.3	73.3	131.3

Power

Percentile	Bench Press	Bench Pull	Right Quad	Left Quad	Right Hamst.	Left Hamst.	Overhead Press	Lat. Pull
1	153	104	102	59	71	66	42	167
5	155	109	110	67	73	71	44	168
10	158	116	119	77	75	77	46	170
15	161	122	123	87	77	83	48	172
20	163	129	126	97	80	89	50	174
25	179	135	129	107	83	93	52	178
30	185	142	132	117	88	95	54	194
35	189	148	135	125	101	97	72	199
40	192	155	138	130	104	99	78	205
45	194	161	162	135	106	101	84	211
50	197	164	171	141	108	103	88	216
55	200	167	180	146	110	105	91	260
60	217	171	189	155	115	110	94	265
65	222	174	198	165	119	116	97	271
70	239	179	248	217	154	136	115	277
75	245	186	257	222	158	142	118	277
80	261	192	266	227	162	148	121	281
85	263	199	275	232	164	154	124	284
90	266	234	284	260	166	187	171	287
95	269	241	293	270	168	193	177	290
99	271	248	301	278	170	198	182	292
Mean	209.5	166.0	185.4	157.3	117.0	117.0	92.8	225.8

APPENDIX XXXIV

Muscular Strength Profile — Males 17-19 Years
Paramount Weight Training Equipment

Percentile	Bench Press	Butterfly	Deltoid	Shoulder Press	Tricep Extension	Bicep Curl
1	80	49	75	48	64	45
5	110	83	90	84	86	48
10	126	89	99	100	94	51
15	140	95	107	106	103	54
20	147	100	113	111	110	57
25	154	111	120	116	116	59
30	162	123	126	122	123	61
35	173	128	131	130	127	67
40	184	132	136	138	130	73
45	189	137	141	144	134	75
50	195	141	145	147	138	77
55	200	146	148	151	141	78
60	206	153	152	154	145	80
65	213	159	156	158	156	82
70	221	166	160	162	167	84
75	228	175	167	169	175	86
80	232	184	175	181	182	89
85	237	193	184	192	190	99
90	241	201	194	203	200	103
95	245	233	222	218	216	106
99	250	250	250	250	250	129
Mean	192.1	146.6	147.9	146.0	146.5	76.7

Percentile	Abdominal	Lower Back	Leg Curl	Leg Extension	Outer Thigh	Inner Thigh
1	48	58	52	84	73	72
5	84	98	69	96	85	83
10	96	108	96	118	96	96
15	108	118	101	128	106	107
20	119	130	106	134	114	117
25	125	140	111	140	122	126
30	128	145	116	153	128	134
35	131	149	121	173	134	142
40	134	154	125	187	140	144
45	137	158	130	192	144	147
50	139	164	135	198	146	149
55	142	175	139	204	148	152
60	146	183	144	212	151	154
65	155	188	149	223	153	156
70	164	194	154	230	156	159
75	172	199	159	233	158	169
80	181	204	164	237	165	182
85	190	220	170	240	175	197
90	202	233	176	243	192	213
95	230	241	181	246	210	229
99	250	250	250	250	239	250
Mean	147.8	170.6	134.4	191.5	146.2	153.4

Muscular Strength Profile — Males 17-19 Years

Percentile	Rotary Right	Torso Left	Lat Pull	Cable Crossover	Hip Flexion Right	Left
1	48	45	56	60	70	70
5	75	66	93	60	71	71
10	94	91	102	61	73	73
15	107	107	110	61	75	75
20	116	116	115	62	77	76
25	124	124	119	63	79	78
30	129	128	123	63	80	80
35	132	132	127	64	82	81
40	136	136	130	69	84	83
45	141	140	134	70	86	85
50	145	144	139	71	88	87
55	153	152	143	72	111	109
60	161	161	147	72	116	114
65	168	168	152	78	122	119
70	175	174	156	79	217	209
75	182	181	162	79	223	214
80	188	187	171	80	228	219
85	196	195	180	81	233	225
90	203	203	192	82	239	229
95	221	221	206	102	244	234
99	250	250	250	104	250	238
Mean	152.2	150.8	146.5	72.2	135.0	130.0

Percentile	Hip Extension Right	Left	Hip Abduction Right	Left	Hip Adduction Right	Left
1	71	71	70	70	85	75
5	75	75	71	71	86	76
10	80	80	73	73	88	78
15	88	85	75	75	89	80
20	107	105	77	76	91	82
25	109	106	79	78	93	83
30	110	108	80	80	94	85
35	112	110	82	81	96	87
40	114	111	84	83	98	89
45	116	113	86	85	99	90
50	118	115	88	87	101	92
55	119	117	129	109	137	131
60	121	118	134	114	141	134
65	123	120	140	119	144	138
70	217	209	145	124	147	141
75	223	214	151	129	151	145
80	228	219	156	134	236	236
85	233	224	233	224	240	239
90	239	229	239	229	243	243
95	244	234	244	234	246	246
99	250	238	250	238	250	250
	148.3	143.3	127.5	122.5	143.7	138.7

APPENDIX XXXV

Muscular Strength Profile — Males 20-29 Years
Paramount Weight Training Equipment

Percentile	Chest Press	Butterfly	Deltoid	Shoulder Press	Tricep Extension	Bicep Curl
1	79	62	66	54	62	31
5	108	95	91	87	97	39
10	128	109	104	99	113	47
15	143	116	114	110	118	51
20	153	120	120	122	122	55
25	163	124	126	127	126	58
30	171	128	132	131	131	62
35	178	133	139	135	136	66
40	185	144	148	139	142	70
45	195	154	154	143	149	75
50	208	161	161	150	156	79
55	218	168	168	160	166	83
60	225	174	174	170	174	87
65	232	178	180	181	180	91
70	239	182	185	190	185	95
75	242	186	190	196	191	100
80	243	190	199	202	201	106
85	245	204	208	211	213	111
90	246	223	225	229	230	119
95	248	238	238	239	240	130
99	250	250	250	250	250	183
Mean	200.4	160.0	161.0	161.1	161.8	83.0

Percentile	Abdominal	Lower Back	Leg Curl	Leg Extension	Outer Thigh	Inner Thigh
1	72	88	61	42	61	49
5	84	107	80	101	80	85
10	97	117	90	120	94	97
15	106	123	97	131	107	113
20	111	129	104	143	121	125
25	117	137	112	156	125	129
30	123	145	119	166	129	133
35	128	156	128	176	133	137
40	133	168	132	190	137	141
45	137	177	138	205	141	145
50	142	184	146	210	146	151
55	146	189	155	216	150	156
60	150	195	159	221	155	161
65	154	201	161	227	161	167
70	158	207	163	230	167	174
75	162	214	166	233	173	181
80	166	227	168	236	180	188
85	173	236	170	240	187	195
90	183	240	172	243	199	203
95	196	245	174	246	209	219
99	219	250	194	250	217	244
Mean	141.8	179.8	139.8	194.9	146.5	154.3

Muscular Strength Profile — Males 20-29 Years

Percentile	Rotary Right	Torso Left	Lat Pull	Hip Flexion Right	Hip Flexion Left
1	64	50	58	85	85
5	95	88	88	89	88
10	109	100	99	94	91
15	117	110	109	99	94
20	122	121	118	104	97
25	127	127	124	109	100
30	132	132	128	114	109
35	140	137	133	119	116
40	148	142	137	122	119
45	156	147	141	125	121
50	162	154	146	129	123
55	169	160	150	132	126
60	174	167	154	138	128
65	179	177	158	141	133
70	184	187	162	146	137
75	189	193	166	151	147
80	198	199	169	155	151
85	209	206	182	160	156
90	233	231	201	165	160
95	241	240	211	240	230
99	250	250	218	250	238
Mean	162.8	161.7	145.8	137.5	132.5

Percentile	Hip Extension Right	Hip Extension Left	Hip Abduction Right	Hip Abduction Left	Hip Adduction Right	Hip Adduction Left
1	71	61	85	75	85	75
5	75	65	87	79	87	79
10	80	70	90	83	90	83
15	86	76	93	88	93	88
20	113	103	96	92	96	94
25	124	114	98	97	98	103
30	134	124	104	101	117	109
35	145	135	112	105	121	113
40	156	146	116	110	125	118
45	181	175	118	114	129	122
50	187	186	120	119	131	127
55	192	196	122	123	133	131
60	215	205	124	126	134	135
65	221	211	126	129	136	139
70	226	216	128	132	138	142
75	232	222	133	135	139	145
80	235	225	142	137	141	148
85	239	229	150	160	143	151
90	242	232	158	169	144	154
95	246	236	226	226	226	226
99	250	239	233	233	233	233
Mean	173.3	168.3	131.8	126.3	135.0	129.5

APPENDIX XXXVI

Muscular Strength Profile — Males 30-39 Years
Paramount Weight Training Equipment

Percentile	Chest Press	Butterfly	Deltoid	Shoulder Press	Tricep Extension	Bicep Curl
1	117	86	87	86	76	45
5	129	93	96	90	84	47
10	156	118	107	96	94	50
15	170	124	114	103	112	52
20	177	130	118	119	128	55
25	183	136	122	128	132	57
30	186	145	126	135	137	60
35	190	151	138	138	142	71
40	193	154	141	142	146	75
45	198	156	144	145	151	82
50	202	159	147	149	155	83
55	207	161	150	152	160	84
60	212	164	153	156	166	85
65	216	166	157	159	172	86
70	221	171	161	163	178	87
75	233	177	164	166	186	88
80	238	182	170	180	195	90
85	241	198	175	198	212	100
90	244	215	183	207	237	102
95	247	241	208	216	243	105
99	250	250	217	246	250	118
Mean	203.5	161.4	145.8	153.0	162.3	80.5

Percentile	Abdominal	Lower Back	Leg Curl	Leg Extension	Outer Thigh	Inner Thigh
1	100	117	110	115	100	100
5	102	142	114	119	103	104
10	104	145	119	124	107	108
15	107	149	124	129	113	116
20	109	152	128	136	127	125
25	111	156	131	143	129	142
30	114	159	135	150	130	144
35	116	163	140	160	132	147
40	130	166	147	174	133	149
45	137	172	153	184	135	151
50	139	179	156	187	138	154
55	141	184	159	191	142	157
60	144	187	162	194	146	160
65	155	191	165	218	154	173
70	157	194	167	237	158	175
75	160	199	170	239	161	177
80	162	204	172	241	173	178
85	174	208	174	243	176	180
90	177	221	177	245	178	182
95	180	235	179	247	182	196
99	188	247	247	250	188	203
Mean	139.2	179.5	153.0	188.8	143.5	152.0

Muscular Strength Profile — Males 30-39 Years

Percentile	Rotary Right	Torso Left	Lat Pull
1	116	116	115
5	120	120	119
10	125	125	122
15	129	129	124
20	133	133	125
25	136	136	126
30	138	138	127
35	140	140	128
40	143	141	129
45	145	143	140
50	151	145	145
55	159	159	154
60	165	165	155
65	170	170	157
70	176	176	158
75	191	191	160
80	194	194	172
85	198	198	183
90	203	203	185
95	209	209	187
99	217	217	189
Mean	160.2	160.0	151.2

APPENDIX XXXVII

Muscular Strength Profile — Males 40-49 Years
Paramount Weight Training Equipment

Percentile	Chest Press	Butterfly	Deltoid	Shoulder Press	Tricep Extension	Bicep Curl
1	85	70	55	56	72	30
5	88	74	59	61	80	33
10	92	78	64	67	86	37
15	95	84	68	72	89	39
20	99	91	73	77	93	41
25	107	93	77	81	97	42
30	116	95	81	85	102	44
35	121	97	86	92	107	45
40	127	99	91	104	115	46
45	134	114	95	110	124	49
50	145	122	100	116	127	57
55	180	130	134	123	130	59
60	185	149	139	129	132	61
65	193	155	143	135	135	64
70	202	158	163	141	140	67
75	207	161	167	147	151	75
80	211	163	172	154	161	87
85	214	166	178	160	172	91
90	218	169	187	166	183	105
95	224	172	196	207	194	112
99	232	174	203	217	202	118
Mean	163.2	125.9	126.6	120.0	127.1	62.1

Percentile	Abdominal	Lower Back	Leg Curl	Leg Extension	Outer Thigh	Inner Thigh
1	85	115	70	67	81	80
5	88	118	74	79	86	82
10	92	121	78	89	92	84
15	94	124	82	96	98	86
20	96	127	86	103	100	89
25	97	129	90	111	102	91
30	99	131	94	118	105	93
35	100	144	98	126	107	101
40	101	151	102	133	110	110
45	104	153	106	142	116	119
50	112	155	110	157	139	129
55	119	157	118	162	142	137
60	122	160	123	167	145	141
65	124	190	127	172	158	146
70	125	193	151	216	161	151
75	127	196	155	231	164	160
80	129	198	159	235	166	169
85	141	199	162	238	168	206
90	145	201	164	242	170	210
95	167	203	167	246	172	215
99	173	204	169	250	174	219
Mean	117.5	163.0	122.1	160.0	132.6	134.2

Muscular Strength Profile — Males 40-49 Years

Percentile	Rotary Right	Torso Left	Lat Pull
1	85	85	86
5	87	87	93
10	90	90	98
15	92	92	100
20	95	95	102
25	98	98	104
30	100	100	106
35	104	104	108
40	109	109	124
45	113	113	128
50	118	118	133
55	131	131	141
60	139	139	161
65	146	146	170
70	154	169	178
75	167	175	184
80	180	182	188
85	188	188	192
90	195	195	196
95	236	236	200
99	250	250	204
Mean	138.4	139.3	143.2

APPENDIX XXXVIII

Muscular Strength Profile — Females 17-19 Years
Paramount Weight Training Equipment

Percentile	Chest Press	Butterfly	Deltoid	Shoulder Press	Tricep Extension	Bicep Curl
1	22	21	25	20	26	4
5	30	25	29	22	34	17
10	38	36	32	24	38	18
15	54	37	33	27	41	20
20	58	38	35	36	43	21
25	61	39	36	38	45	22
30	64	40	37	39	47	23
35	66	42	38	41	50	25
40	67	43	39	42	52	26
45	69	50	48	52	54	27
50	71	53	49	53	56	27
55	72	54	50	54	58	28
60	74	55	52	55	60	29
65	76	57	53	57	63	30
70	79	58	54	58	65	31
75	82	59	64	59	67	32
80	85	70	66	70	70	33
85	99	72	68	72	72	34
90	103	75	79	74	77	44
95	107	87	83	86	82	61
99	119	92	96	92	133	76
Mean	72.3	52.1	54.0	50.7	58.1	29.2

Percentile	Abdominal	Lower Back	Leg Curl	Leg Extension	Outer Thigh	Inner Thigh
1	41	43	23	30	45	43
5	47	59	33	48	67	54
10	52	70	40	54	69	62
15	56	75	48	60	71	66
20	60	80	54	66	74	69
25	62	83	57	72	76	73
30	64	86	61	78	79	76
35	65	89	64	83	82	78
40	67	92	67	89	85	81
45	69	96	70	94	88	83
50	70	100	72	97	92	86
55	78	104	75	101	95	88
60	83	108	79	105	97	91
65	85	111	82	109	100	94
70	87	114	85	113	103	96
75	89	117	90	121	105	99
80	91	121	94	131	108	114
85	94	128	100	140	113	118
90	98	135	108	148	117	122
95	102	152	119	155	124	131
99	123	161	127	229	163	150
Mean	76.3	101.2	74.1	103.1	91.0	90.4

Muscular Strength Profile — Females 17-19 Years

Percentile	Rotary Right	Torso Left	Lat Pull	Cable Crossover	Hip Flexion Right	Left
1	31	30	20	20	26	26
5	41	39	33	20	31	31
10	46	42	36	21	38	37
15	50	46	39	21	64	62
20	54	49	50	22	91	74
25	57	52	53	23	93	78
30	59	54	55	23	95	82
35	62	57	66	36	98	86
40	65	59	67	36	100	91
45	68	62	68	37	102	95
50	72	65	70	38	104	99
55	78	68	71	38	106	103
60	83	72	72	39	109	107
65	86	74	73	39	113	111
70	88	77	81	56	116	115
75	91	80	84	57	119	119
80	94	82	86	57	123	124
85	97	98	88	58	150	136
90	106	104	90	58	176	165
95	116	112	93	59	183	177
99	156	133	98	60	188	187
Mean	69.8	70.0	67.5	40.0	106.5	102.3

Percentile	Hip Extension Right	Left	Hip Abduction Right	Left	Hip Adduction Right	Left
1	26	26	27	17	27	17
5	30	30	35	25	35	25
10	35	35	41	31	41	31
15	40	40	44	34	44	34
20	67	48	48	38	48	38
25	83	64	52	42	52	42
30	99	99	62	52	70	66
35	105	104	73	63	76	71
40	108	107	80	83	80	75
45	111	110	84	86	84	78
50	114	112	88	89	88	82
55	117	115	91	91	91	93
60	120	117	96	94	100	100
65	125	120	101	98	111	105
70	130	126	108	104	122	124
75	135	142	119	109	133	129
80	140	157	130	133	136	135
85	153	173	141	139	140	139
90	169	204	149	142	143	142
95	204	212	154	146	149	146
99	216	218	158	149	157	149
Mean	111.5	113.4	89.6	84.6	92.5	87.5

APPENDIX XXXIX

Muscular Strength Profile — Females 20-29 Years
Paramount Weight Training Equipment

Percentile	Chest Press	Butterfly	Deltoid	Shoulder Press	Tricep Extension	Bicep Curl
1	25	25	25	20	26	3
5	29	29	29	23	34	15
10	34	34	33	27	39	16
15	38	35	37	30	42	17
20	42	37	39	32	45	18
25	45	38	41	34	47	19
30	47	40	43	36	50	20
35	50	41	45	38	52	21
40	53	52	46	39	55	22
45	56	53	48	41	57	23
50	59	55	50	54	60	24
55	61	57	53	56	62	25
60	64	58	55	58	65	26
65	67	60	57	60	68	27
70	70	62	60	62	72	28
75	75	64	62	65	75	29
80	80	66	66	69	79	33
85	86	68	70	73	85	39
90	95	81	74	79	90	42
95	109	97	88	88	102	53
99	140	108	138	115	131	71
Mean	69.8	55.5	52.2	52.8	60.3	29.3

Percentile	Abdominal	Lower Back	Leg Curl	Leg Extension	Outer Thigh	Inner Thigh
1	33	41	28	27	41	23
5	42	49	37	37	47	41
10	49	57	43	48	54	52
15	52	61	49	52	58	58
20	55	66	54	55	62	64
25	58	71	59	59	65	68
30	61	76	62	62	68	70
35	63	82	66	66	72	72
40	65	86	69	70	76	74
45	67	89	72	80	81	76
50	70	92	76	91	86	78
55	72	95	81	96	90	80
60	74	99	85	101	93	82
65	77	103	92	106	96	84
70	79	108	99	111	98	88
75	81	113	103	118	101	93
80	84	121	107	129	104	98
85	101	129	112	140	110	102
90	106	145	124	151	118	117
95	114	158	134	184	131	131
99	120	180	146	234	188	181
Mean	74.4	102.9	31.3	97.7	89.2	84.0

Muscular Strength Profile — Females 20-29 Years

Percentile	Rotary Right	Torso Left	Lat Pull	Hip Flexion Right	Hip Flexion Left	Cable Crossover
1	29	15	40	41	41	20
5	39	29	42	45	45	22
10	42	32	45	51	51	24
15	45	36	48	57	57	26
20	47	39	51	66	66	28
25	50	42	53	75	75	30
30	53	45	56	85	85	38
35	56	48	58	91	91	39
40	59	51	61	95	94	40
45	62	55	62	99	98	41
50	65	58	64	103	101	42
55	68	61	66	111	105	43
60	71	64	68	123	113	45
65	74	68	70	129	122	47
70	76	71	82	135	129	49
75	80	75	85	141	136	57
80	85	80	89	148	143	59
85	90	85	92	155	150	61
90	98	93	98	168	160	75
95	116	119	118	182	176	77
99	144	140	135	199	199	79
Mean	66.1	66.0	70.0	110.2	105.2	45.7

Percentile	Hip Extension Right	Hip Extension Left	Hip Abduction Right	Hip Abduction Left	Hip Adduction Right	Hip Adduction Left
1	41	31	40	30	41	31
5	45	37	43	33	45	37
10	51	44	46	37	51	44
15	57	52	49	41	57	51
20	69	65	52	45	62	55
25	83	75	56	52	66	59
30	88	80	59	58	70	63
35	93	86	63	64	74	67
40	98	91	67	70	78	71
45	125	102	72	75	83	78
50	131	122	85	94	92	87
55	136	129	97	103	101	96
60	142	137	116	111	108	105
65	150	146	121	118	116	114
70	159	155	126	125	123	118
75	169	165	131	134	128	122
80	181	178	138	143	133	126
85	193	190	144	152	138	130
90	205	203	157	162	143	134
95	238	231	177	176	158	169
99	250	250	187	187	242	232
Mean	130.0	122.9	100.5	95.5	99.1	93.8

APPENDIX XXXX

Muscular Strength Profile — Females 30-39 Years
Paramount Weight Training Equipment

Percentile	Chest Press	Butterfly	Deltoid	Shoulder Press	Tricep Extension	Bicep Curl
1	26	25	2	25	27	20
5	31	28	20	29	34	20
10	37	37	22	34	37	20
15	43	37	25	35	39	20
20	48	38	27	36	41	21
25	53	39	29	37	52	21
30	56	40	31	38	54	21
35	57	41	34	39	55	22
40	59	41	36	40	56	22
45	61	42	38	41	58	27
50	63	49	41	43	59	27
55	64	50	46	52	61	28
60	66	51	50	55	63	28
65	68	52	53	57	65	28
70	69	53	57	60	67	29
75	77	54	60	65	69	29
80	85	67	64	81	82	30
85	90	69	67	89	97	38
90	95	70	83	100	101	43
95	104	72	93	107	104	44
99	169	83	98	113	112	44
Mean	73.0	50.1	48.8	56.4	64.3	28.1

Percentile	Abdominal	Lower Back	Leg Curl	Leg Extension	Outer Thigh	Inner Thigh
1	28	40	41	40	41	55
5	38	44	47	43	45	57
10	46	49	52	46	51	59
15	49	54	57	50	56	61
20	51	59	62	53	68	63
25	54	65	67	56	69	65
30	67	70	69	59	71	68
35	68	76	70	62	73	70
40	69	81	72	65	74	72
45	71	88	74	68	76	74
50	72	91	76	72	78	77
55	73	95	78	75	80	79
60	74	100	80	79	83	82
65	75	105	82	82	95	84
70	77	110	83	90	97	98
75	79	118	91	103	100	103
80	81	123	98	107	103	107
85	86	131	103	112	115	111
90	102	146	110	127	119	116
95	121	191	118	155	124	136
99	128	214	127	185	128	157
Mean	72.0	97.1	78.9	87.1	84.6	84.4

Muscular Strength Profile — Females 30-39 Years

Percentile	Rotary Right	Torso Left	Lat Pull
1	21	28	27
5	26	37	46
10	32	39	49
15	35	42	52
20	38	44	54
25	41	46	67
30	44	48	68
35	48	51	70
40	49	53	71
45	51	56	72
50	54	59	74
55	56	61	75
60	59	63	76
65	61	65	78
70	63	67	81
75	65	69	84
80	68	71	86
85	95	97	100
90	102	104	104
95	112	125	108
99	141	141	127
Mean	61.8	63.9	74.3

APPENDIX XXXXI

Muscular Strength Profile — Females 40-49 Years
Paramount Weight Training Equipment

Percentile	Chest Press	Butterfly	Deltoid	Shoulder Press	Tricep Extension	Bicep Curl
1	25	25	10	25	25	20
5	27	25	12	25	26	20
10	38	26	14	25	28	20
15	39	26	24	26	29	20
20	40	27	24	26	37	20
25	41	27	25	27	38	20
30	41	37	26	27	38	21
35	42	37	26	27	39	21
40	49	37	27	28	40	21
45	51	38	28	28	41	21
50	52	38	30	29	42	21
55	53	38	32	38	49	28
60	54	39	39	41	50	28
65	55	39	39	48	51	28
70	56	39	39	50	52	28
75	57	43	43	52	53	29
80	60	45	45	53	54	29
85	66	52	51	55	69	29
90	67	53	52	56	72	29
95	68	54	53	67	81	38
99	69	54	54	69	84	39
Mean	50.9	39.0	33.8	38.1	48.1	25.4

Percentile	Abdominal	Lower Back	Leg Curl	Leg Extension	Outer Thigh	Inner Thigh
1	40	40	20	25	40	40
5	40	41	23	28	42	42
10	41	43	46	37	44	44
15	41	44	47	40	67	54
20	42	64	48	49	67	55
25	43	66	49	50	67	56
30	43	67	50	50	68	57
35	44	69	52	51	68	67
40	54	82	55	52	68	67
45	55	83	58	53	68	68
50	56	84	60	54	69	68
55	67	85	62	67	69	69
60	67	85	64	68	69	69
65	68	86	65	70	70	70
70	69	87	67	72	70	70
75	70	94	69	79	70	71
80	71	95	71	80	70	80
85	77	96	79	81	71	81
90	80	97	81	92	80	82
95	82	98	83	93	82	83
99	84	99	84	94	84	84
Mean	58.6	78.7	59.0	61.8	68.3	66.6

Muscular Strength Profile — Females 40-49 Years

Percentile	Rotary Right	Torso Left	Lat Pull
1	25	25	30
5	27	28	32
10	38	36	34
15	39	37	54
20	41	39	54
25	42	40	55
30	52	52	55
35	52	53	56
40	53	54	56
45	53	54	56
50	54	55	57
55	54	55	57
60	55	56	58
65	55	57	66
70	56	57	67
75	65	69	67
80	66	71	68
85	67	72	68
90	68	74	69
95	69	76	69
99	69	79	69
Mean	53.6	54.5	58.5

CARDIOVASCULAR EXERCISE LOG

Date	Activity	Distance	Time

CARDIOVASCULAR EXERCISE LOG

Date	Activity	Distance	Time

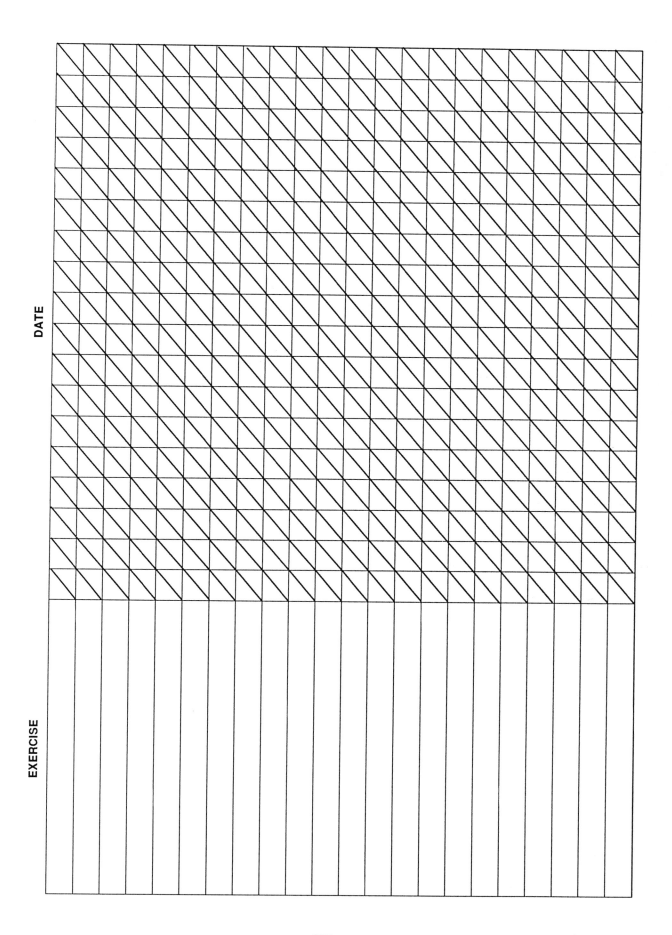

DATE

EXERCISE

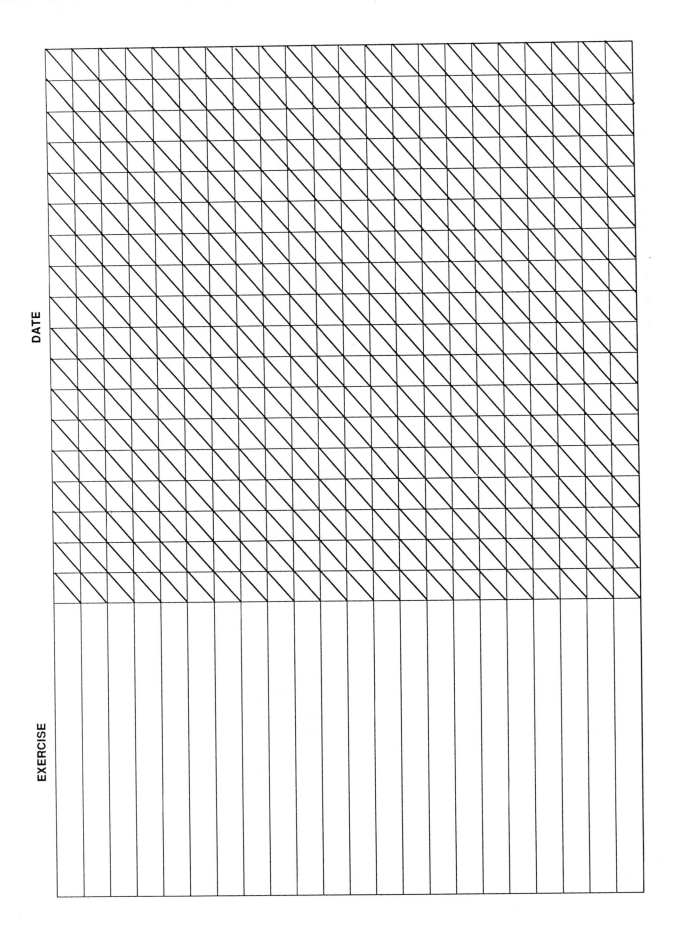

DATE

EXERCISE

INDEX